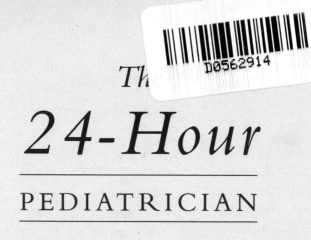

The
24-Hour

PEDIATRICIAN

The
24-Hour

PEDIATRICIAN

DOCTORS FROM
80 LEADING CHILDREN'S HOSPITALS
OFFER PARENTS THEIR BEST TIPS
FOR MAKING KIDS
FEEL BETTER FASTER

CHRISTINA ELSTON

 THREE RIVERS PRESS
NEW YORK

Author's Note

No book, including this one, can ever replace a consultation with a doctor or other health professional. I've written it to help you work more effectively with your pediatrician. Please share it with your doctor to help you both make the best health-care choices for your child.

Published by Three Rivers Press, New York, New York.
Member of the Crown Publishing Group, a division of
Random House, Inc.
www.randomhouse.com

THREE RIVERS PRESS and the Tugboat design are registered trademarks of Random House, Inc.

Printed in the United States of America
Design by Meryl Sussman Levavi/Digitext

Library of Congress Cataloging-in-Publication Data
Elston, Christina.
The 24-hour pediatrician : doctors from 80 leading children's hospitals offer parents their best tips for making kids feel better / Christina Elston.
p.;   cm.
1. Pediatrics.   2. Children—Diseases—Diagnosis.   3. Diagnosis, Differential.   I. Title: Twenty-four-hour pediatrician.   II. Title
RJ45 .E56 2002
618.92—dc21   2002018814

ISBN 0-8129-3134-3

10 9 8 7 6 5 4 3 2 1

First Edition

To my family, who can always make it better.

Acknowledgments

Special thanks to:

All of the doctors who offered me their time and knowledge.

The hospital publicists who helped me find those doctors.

Betsy Amster, who believed in my idea.

Elizabeth Rapoport, whose editing made this book what it is.

Stephanie Higgs, for her guidance and support.

Niceole Levy, Lolita Harper, and Angela Smith, for their assistance.

Michael Evanston, for lending his artistic talent.

My mom, for her inspiration.

Contents

Introduction

The idea for this book basically came from my mom. When I was growing up, she had some remedies up her sleeve that seemed to me part medicine, part love, and part magic. When my brother or I had a cold we got 7UP and buttered toast, a special bed on the couch, and free run of the afternoon cartoons to keep us quiet. If we had a cut or scrape, Mom applied an antiseptic she called the "red badge of courage," followed by a bandage and a kiss. For bumps and bruises, we got to sit in her lap and be hugged and rocked while she held an ice-filled plastic bag, wrapped in a wet washcloth, to the spot. And while we were getting better, we *felt* better!

Along with Mom's maternal instincts, she had a good old-fashioned family doctor to rely on. He was the kind of guy who didn't have to look at your chart to know your name. He was my mom's doctor, delivered my brother and me, and took care of the whole family for several years. He gave advice over the phone and treated the whole bunch of us in one visit if we were sharing that year's brand of winter flu. Visits lasted at least half an hour, so he had time to tell us little things like what not to eat if we had an upset stomach, or that warm towels would help an earache until the prescription kicked in.

When I became a mother, I still had Mom to call on (long-distance) when my daughter got sick, but I found myself with an HMO that had no time for advice instead of a family doctor who knew my children's names. I took to researching health questions myself. But the books often gave conflicting advice, forcing me to guess which one to follow.

Then I took over the children's health column at a parenting magazine and felt like I had hit the jackpot. At last I could ask several doctors about the same topic and gather a consensus opinion. Plus, a thirty-minute interview rather than a hurried ten-minute office visit gave me time to learn the extras that can make a big difference. The column began to mirror whatever nagging questions I had about my daughter's childhood ailments, and I thought that it was too bad other parents couldn't do what I was doing. That's where this book comes in.

Here you'll find sound medical information about basic children's health issues—plus the TLC every doctor would prescribe if he or she had the time. I spoke with six to ten different doctors from leading children's hospitals across the country to get the best make-it-feel-better advice for kids' most common ailments. These are people who devote themselves specifically to children's health. Most of them have many years of experience dealing with kids and their parents, so they were more than ready for my questions. Beyond the basic medical advice, I've gathered doctors' favorite tricks and tips for making kids *feel better,* not just curing their ailment. I asked them to tell me the things they wished they had time to tell all the parents who come to see them, and they were more than generous with their time and knowledge.

I sometimes got conflicting advice from these medical professionals, but when that happened, I made sure to let you, the reader, know about it. Different approaches work best for different kids; your own pediatrician can offer further advice. This book isn't a substitute for a doctor's care, but a supplement. I hope it will help you and your doctor keep your child happy and healthy. The doctors here (along with your own) can offer medical information, and sometimes a little magic. You add the love and make it better.

The
24-Hour

PEDIATRICIAN

Choosing a Pediatrician

There was a time when one doctor took care of the whole family. He or she treated Mom and Dad's minor illnesses, watched over Mom through her pregnancies, delivered the babies, and took care of the kids as well. But as our knowledge about children's health has changed, so have the doctors.

Pediatricians today must take three or more years of courses *after* medical school to become trained in pediatrics. Then, to become board-certified, they must pass a detailed test given by the American Board of Pediatrics. This helps qualify them to look after the unique health-care needs of children, including growth and development, behavior and learning issues, nutrition, and immunizations, as well as illnesses and injuries. A good pediatrician should be able to address your child's health needs from infancy through puberty, and know to refer you to a specialist for complex problems.

WHEN TO START LOOKING

Whether you're having your first baby and have never had a pediatrician before, or are moving or changing insurance providers and have to give up your current pediatrician, the time to start looking for a doctor for your child is now. The American Academy of Pediatrics and most doctors advise parents not to wait until their child is ill or needs a checkup before looking for a pediatrician.

Some doctors say that the ideal time to start looking for your very first pediatrician, is before you even get pregnant. Others say that you should start about three months before the baby is expected—keeping in mind that sometimes babies come early. In any case, you should give yourself enough time to interview several doctors.

> By the sixth month, if you've had an ultrasound, you might even know about potential problems with the baby. If this is the case, you can look for a pediatrician who has a special interest in this area.
> —WILLIAM G. BITHONEY, M.D.,
> ST. JOSEPH'S CHILDREN'S HOSPITAL, NEW JERSEY

WHERE TO LOOK

If you're part of a managed-care program, you'll have to get information on which pediatricians are available through your health-insurance provider. Otherwise, call your nearest university medical school or local children's hospital for referrals, or network with friends and coworkers for their suggestions. Your family physician or obstetrician can be a good source of information.

To get a good referral, call your local academic center and speak with the chief resident. The chief resident will often know which doctors are especially good.
—WILLIAM G. BITHONEY, M.D.,
ST. JOSEPH'S CHILDREN'S HOSPITAL, NEW JERSEY

The best and most objective measure of a pediatrician, according to many doctors, is board certification by the American Academy of Pediatrics. Board-certified doctors append F.A.A.P. (Fellow, American Academy of Pediatrics) to their titles and have to renew their training every seven years, so they keep up on new information and techniques. Otherwise, doctors don't often change their practice techniques.

If you're getting a referral from a friend or coworker, find out if the doctor and office staff are good at handling questions, and whether telephone calls and emergencies are managed well. How long is the wait in the office for a scheduled appointment? Ask if the children seem to like the doctor, and whether she seems to relate well to children as well as parents. You might also want to ask if there is anything about the pediatrician or office that has ever bothered your friend.

Once you've compiled a list of potential candidates, you'll need to contact their offices to ask a few questions, and to set up in-person interviews with any who seem promising. This way you can check out the office environment and make sure the chemistry is right. Doctors say that it's not a good idea to bring children on this visit. You and the doctor will both be better able to concentrate, and to speak freely, if you aren't distracted by children.

WHAT TO ASK

The main reason to sit down and talk with doctors you are considering, rather than doing interviews over the phone, is to make sure that the "chemistry" is right—especially with the parent who will have the primary responsibility for bringing the child to the doctor. Ideally, you'll find a pediatrician whose personality is compatible with yours, someone you would be happy to work with.

> More important than the doctor's views on issues that might cause controversy (such as circumcision, breast-feeding, or use of antibiotics) is the doctor's attitude. You want a doctor who exhibits a certain degree of flexibility and doesn't mind explaining his views.
> —EDWARD R. B. McCABE, M.D., PH.D.,
> MATTEL CHILDREN'S HOSPITAL AT UCLA

Prepare a list of questions in advance, bring them with you, and be ready to take notes. Doctors recommend discussing topics like an interest in alternative medicine, or religious objections, with any physician you are considering. Find out how long the doctor has been in practice. How long has the staff been with him or her? A doctor who has long-term relationships with staff probably has a better-run operation than one with constant turnover.

> This is someone who is going to be a partner with you in keeping your child healthy. It's important that you trust your pediatrician, because then you are more likely to follow his or her instructions.
> —LINDA McCABE, PH.D., UCLA

OFFICE LOCATION AND HOURS

Find out if the doctor is convenient for you. The doctor's office should be close enough to home that you can take your child in for checkups and get there quickly if your child is ill. If it's difficult for you to get your child to the doctor during business hours, you'll want to find someone who takes evening or weekend appointments at least occasionally. Ask how long it generally takes to get an appointment with the doctor. Many pediatricians don't keep their own schedules, so you'll need to ask the office staff about this.

> If you have a special interest, such as holistic medicine, find out how any doctor you're considering feels about it. Also, find out about any special areas of interest the doctor might have. Sometimes even a doctor who isn't a sub-specialist knows a lot about a particular area, such as allergy and immunology. If you know your child has a particular health problem, it's a good idea to find a doctor who has taken a special interest in that area.
>
> —RACHELLE TYLER, M.D., M.P.H.,
> MATTEL CHILDREN'S HOSPITAL AT UCLA

It's also important to know what will happen when the doctor is on vacation or otherwise unavailable. Is it a group practice, with more than one physician? Who will you see if you can't see your doctor? All doctors need some sort of cross-coverage arrangement so that they have time to lead personal lives and to renew their training when they need to.

OFFICE ENVIRONMENT

The pediatrician's office should be both child-friendly and child-safe. The colors and artwork on the wall should be appealing to children. There should be games and toys for them to play with and/or videos for them to watch. Look for a warm, welcoming, well-lit environment and a responsive and friendly office staff.

When you visit the office, keep in mind that most pediatricians' offices will be a bit hectic. Some will have times of the day when the doctor sees sick children as opposed to well children. Others might have a separate alcove in the waiting room for sick children, or make it a practice to take sick children straight into an examining room. They should have some system for keeping them separated, though this can be challenging.

—EDWARD R. B. MCCABE, M.D., PH.D.,
MATTEL CHILDREN'S HOSPITAL AT UCLA

The exam room itself should be friendly, and it's a nice idea if there are gowns readily accessible for older children who need to undress. Each exam room should have a sink for washing hands, and the tables should be safe and well padded, with paper that is easy to change.

There should be a place in each exam room for you to sit if the doctor needs to talk with you. It's also a good idea for the pediatrician to have a separate consultation room, so there's a comfortable place to have a longer discussion if necessary.

Check out the bathrooms. Are they clean and kid-friendly?

IN AN EMERGENCY

Ask about how the office handles emergencies. Some doctors use a telephone triage service, where parents can call at any time and talk to a nurse or other health-care professional about their child. The triage worker will ask questions to help determine whether the child needs to come into the office or go to a hospital or urgent-care center. Doctors say that some of these services can be quite helpful, and of good quality, giving parents a twenty-four-hour resource. If the doctor doesn't use telephone triage, ask whether she or a colleague is available to speak with you in an emergency. In either case, a good pediatrician should have some way to answer emergency calls, even at night. If the doctor uses an answering service, how quickly will your calls be returned?

Does the doctor use an urgent-care center that might take care of emergency visits? These centers are generally set up to handle emergencies or evening and weekend visits without exposing your child to a hospital's emergency room. Knowing the protocol beforehand might save you from being kept on hold if you call the doctor's office.

If your child has to be hospitalized, you'll want to know if your pediatrician will meet you in the emergency room. Doctors say that if the pediatrician uses a community hospital rather than a children's hospital, he or she should be prepared to meet you in the emergency room, because community hospitals aren't as experienced at treating children. However, if your doctor uses a children's hospital, a visit from him or her isn't really necessary.

HOSPITAL PRIVILEGES

Most doctors have "privileges"—the right to practice—at one or more hospitals in their area. Find out where the doctors you are considering have privileges, especially if you're pregnant. If your pediatrician doesn't have privileges at the hospital where you will deliver your baby, he or she won't be able to come and examine your baby before you leave the hospital. The pediatrician also won't be able to care for your infant in the well-baby nursery.

Find out if the doctor does in-patient coverage in the hospital, or whether he or she has a hospitalist (a doctor who handles patient loads at that particular hospital) do that. This is controversial. Hospitalists at a children's hospital give very good care, and there are advantages to having someone who is located on the hospital premises all the time. However, some doctors are concerned that the continuity of care might be interrupted if the child is handed off to a hospitalist. If your doctor doesn't do his or her own in-patient care, decide whether you are comfortable with this.

> Ideally, it's best to have a pediatrician who is affiliated with a children's hospital, because children's hospitals are better prepared to treat children than community hospitals. However, if you've got a good board-certified pediatrician who will know if your child needs to be transferred to a children's hospital, you'll be fine.
>
> —WILLIAM G. BITHONEY, M.D.,
> ST. JOSEPH'S CHILDREN'S HOSPITAL, NEW JERSEY

WORKING TOGETHER

Once you've found a pediatrician with whom both you and your child are comfortable, you can focus on working together to keep your child healthy. Your part of the bargain, according to doctors, is to be well prepared when making calls or coming in for office visits, and to help prepare your child as well.

If your child is old enough, talk with him about visits to the doctor. Let your child know that the doctor is there to keep him healthy, or to help him feel better if he's sick; don't ever threaten that a doctor will give your child a shot if he isn't good. If you know what's going to happen at the visit (such as whether he's going to get an immunization), prepare him for that as well. Read related books and play with toys to help your child get ready for upcoming visits.

While in the office, be supportive and involved in helping your child through the experience. Also, support
decisions and treatment even if your child resists.
Don't argue with the doctor in front of your child about
whether a certain procedure is necessary.

—RACHELLE TYLER, M.D., M.P.H.,
MATTEL CHILDREN'S HOSPITAL AT UCLA

If your child is ill, you might sometimes have an idea
about what might be wrong or how your child should be
treated. Maybe you're convinced that antibiotics are necessary or that your child needs a prescription cough syrup.
Doctors advise that you hear what your pediatrician has to
say before bringing up your own ideas. Of course you should
feel free to ask questions and discuss your child's treatment,
but in the end you need to trust your doctor.

Try to prioritize your list of questions. Some pediatricians are only able to spend an average of about six
minutes per office visit, so you might not get them all
answered. Identify the four to six that are most important to you.

—EDWARD R. B. MCCABE, M.D., PH.D.,
MATTEL CHILDREN'S HOSPITAL AT UCLA

Some pediatricians are now answering patients' questions
via e-mail. Ask whether your doctor does this. There may
also be a child health associate or pediatric nurse practitioner
in the doctor's office who can help.

If you ever become frustrated with your pediatrician,
try to determine whether there's a pattern of unsatisfactory
behavior or whether the doctor might be focusing on a very
ill child in the next room whose case he is trying to figure
out. If you have ongoing concerns that the doctor doesn't
address, it might be time to find a new pediatrician.

CALLING WITH QUESTIONS

No matter how healthy your child might be, you will eventually need to call your pediatrician's office with a question. Find out if your doctor sets aside a call-in hour when parents can call without interrupting the doctor's patient visits. This way you can make nonemergency calls at the time most convenient for the doctor.

> Call as soon as you believe you have something to call about. Don't stew all evening about whether or not to call about your child's fever and then finally decide to do it at three A.M. If you're calling about a condition that has been going on for weeks and months, and not an emergency, call during your pediatrician's regular call-in hours.
>
> —WILLIAM G. BITHONEY, M.D.,
> ST. JOSEPH'S CHILDREN'S HOSPITAL, NEW JERSEY

When calling your doctor's office with a question, be prepared to provide your child's name, date of birth, office or medical record number if you have it, allergies, chronic conditions, recent hospitalizations and illnesses, and a list of any medications your child is taking. Keep all this information near the phone for when you need to call.

Before calling your doctor with a minor health matter, also have handy:

- What and how severe your child's symptoms are
- Whether your child has a fever, and how high it is
- How long your child has been ill
- Whether your child is breathing normally
- Whether your child is urinating and having bowel movements as normal
- If your child's appetite is normal

- If your child's activity level is normal
- Whether you've given your child any medication, prescription or over-the-counter, and whether it has helped
- Any other measures you might have taken to help (e.g., sponge baths for a fever)
- Whether your child might have been exposed to an infectious illness
- If you've recently traveled or had guests from out of the country
- Whether your child's immunizations are up to date
- Changes in feeding or new foods introduced
- What exactly prompted the call (maybe your child has been sick all week, but something specific has just happened that made you decide to call the doctor)

You should also make a list of questions that you want the doctor to answer, so you don't forget something and have to call back.

Allergies

With symptoms that range from mild seasonal sniffles to severe breathing problems, or a rash that covers the body, allergies can be a minor annoyance or a life-threatening danger. But even at their most minor, doctors say that allergies—whether they be to a food, pollen, mold, dust, or pet dander—should be treated. "There are too many people who think that going around with a runny nose is just part of being a kid," says Stuart Abramson, M.D., Ph.D., of Texas Children's Hospital.

Even relatively minor allergies that go untreated can cause significant problems. A child who is constantly taking over-the-counter medications that cause drowsiness might have difficulty concentrating in school, and her grades might suffer. Kids with chronic congestion also might "mouth breathe," which can cause an overbite to form.

Recurrent ear infections, sinusitis, and sleep apnea might all be signs that your child has an allergy. Get an allergy evaluation before considering ear tubes or adenoid removal for these problems.

—STUART ABRAMSON, M.D., PH.D.,
TEXAS CHILDREN'S HOSPITAL

Children can develop allergies from the time they are infants, with food allergies showing up earliest in life. As children start to get older, sensitivity to airborne allergens can develop, often sensitivity to indoor allergens such as dust mites or pet dander. Children usually don't show sensitivity to outdoor allergens such as pollen before the age of three to five.

If you have a history of allergy in the immediate family, your child is likely to develop them as well. About 10 percent of children who have no family history of allergy will still be allergic during their lifetime, while 40 percent of children who have one parent with allergies will be allergic, Abramson says. Parents' specific allergies are not necessarily passed on. It is just the tendency to react allergically that is passed on. So while you might be allergic to peanuts, it could be pollen that bothers your child.

Allergies—even to pollens—can happen at any time of year, so don't assume that because your child's symptoms don't occur during spring or summer that they are not due to allergies.

—ANDREA MCCOY, M.D.,
TEMPLE UNIVERSITY CHILDREN'S MEDICAL CENTER,
PHILADELPHIA, PENNSYLVANIA

Allergies usually cause thin, clear, runny nose, itchy nose or eyes, but no fever. Some children might also have fatigue and loss of appetite along with these symptoms. Unlike with a cold or virus, symptoms persist well beyond three weeks.

Usually, children with allergies don't have much of a cough, but they can get "allergic shiners," discoloration under the eye that often comes from rubbing. Children can also get hives or rash if they come in contact with an allergen.

FIRST RESPONSE

ELIMINATE THE ALLERGEN

The best way to help your child avoid allergic reactions is, of course, to keep him away from the things he is allergic to. Sometimes it's easy to tell what those things are. You might notice that your child has symptoms around animals at a certain time of year, or when she eats a certain food. This means you can help avoid the food or animals, or give your child a prescription allergy medication when the pollens that bother your child are in the air.

Sometimes, however, a child's allergies aren't readily apparent. If you can't figure out what your child is allergic to, see your pediatrician and get a referral to an allergist, who can test your child and find out exactly what she is sensitive to. Testing is also helpful if you suspect that your child is allergic to animal dander, but want to be sure before considering saying goodbye to a beloved pet.

Two common kinds of allergy testing are prick puncture testing (scratch testing), which involves placing small amounts of an allergen on the skin and then scratching or puncturing the skin, and intradermal testing, where a small amount of the allergen is injected superficially under the skin.

"Most people have the misconception that allergy testing is extremely painful, or that they will have to keep coming back to the allergist for visit after visit before they know what they are allergic to," says Robert Feldman, M.D., of Children's

Hospital of New York. In fact, the testing causes just mild discomfort, and most people's allergies can be identified in just a visit or two, Feldman says.

> Have the doctor perform a test on you first. Then you can tell your child exactly how it feels. Your child is more likely to believe you than to trust a doctor he or she has never met before. And if your child sees you react calmly to the test, it will help her feel more confident.
>
> —ROBERT FELDMAN, M.D.,
> CHILDREN'S HOSPITAL OF NEW YORK

Though the testing itself isn't very painful, the idea of it might upset your child. Your attitude toward the testing can make a big difference. Talk with your child about his allergic symptoms, and the problems they cause, and explain that by getting these tests and finding out what he is allergic to, the doctor can help control the symptoms. You can also explain that it's not as bad as getting a shot, and that it is more of a scratch than a stick.

Doctors generally prefer not to do scratch testing on children younger than two or three. Another type of testing is the RAST test, a blood test used to determine the level of antibodies in the blood, which shows whether or not a person is allergic. This test is much quicker and easier for the child, but is more expensive than scratch or intradermal testing.

COMFORT CARE

Once you know what your child is allergic to, you can take steps to minimize how much or how often she is exposed to those things. Your doctor can also prescribe some medications that might help.

AIRBORNE ALLERGIES

Using a HEPA (High Efficiency Particle Arresting) filter on your vacuum can help reduce the level of allergens in your home. HEPA room filters, however, are not worth the cost, says Stuart Abramson, M.D., Ph.D., of Texas Children's Hospital. These devices only filter particles out of the air, but won't pick up particles from surfaces, where allergens tend to cling.

> When trying to reduce allergens such as dust, pollen, or pet dander in your home, focus on your child's bedroom. We spend one-third of our time in bed, so it's important that this room be as free of allergens as possible.
>
> —STUART ABRAMSON, M.D., PH.D.,
> TEXAS CHILDREN'S HOSPITAL

If your child has been exposed to pollen or pet dander that she is sensitive to, have her take a cool shower or bath and change clothes, or at least wash her hands and face to get as much of the allergen off as possible. You can use cool compresses to help with itchy eyes, and even give a dose of over-the-counter antihistamines as directed as long as you are using it for an isolated incident, and she is not already taking prescription allergy medication.

Over-the-counter antihistamines might make your child sleepy or hyper, so be aware of the time of day and how your child generally reacts to the medication before you give it. Don't try an antihistamine for the first time right before school, or right before your child is going to bed. Find out what side effects she experiences first.

Prescription allergy medications are generally nondrowsy and easy for children to take. Most are taken just once or twice a day, unlike over-the-counter medications, which often must be taken three or four times a day. In addition, over-the-counter medications tend to lose a bit of their effectiveness over time, less likely with prescription medications.

FOOD ALLERGIES

If your child has a food allergy, doctors stress that you have to begin educating your child about the allergy as soon as he is old enough to understand. Even before children can talk, you can show them foods they cannot eat and say "no."

> Teach your child not to hide anything about the fact that she is allergic. Some children try to because they don't want to be "different," but this can be dangerous.
>
> —ROBERT FELDMAN, M.D.,
> CHILDREN'S HOSPITAL OF NEW YORK

> If your child is seven or older, have him talk with his class about his food allergy. This way, everyone knows about it upfront, and your child won't have to explain it over and over to individual classmates.
>
> —ANDREA McCOY, M.D.,
> TEMPLE UNIVERSITY CHILDREN'S MEDICAL CENTER,
> PHILADELPHIA, PENNSYLVANIA

If your child's food allergy is severe, a reaction could be life-threatening. For this reason, you need to talk about the allergy with anyone who will be caring for your child—including relatives, baby-sitters, teachers, and other caregivers, or the parents of your child's friends. Explain to them precisely what foods your child is allergic to, and that these foods might be present in prepared foods that you wouldn't expect would have them, for example, ground nuts in a chocolate cake mix.

If you have a child with a food allergy, try to focus on the things they *can* eat, rather than always talking about the things they *can't*. Pack your child's own goodies for school parties or outings with friends, so that she isn't left out at snack time.

—ANDREA McCOY, M.D.,
TEMPLE UNIVERSITY CHILDREN'S MEDICAL CENTER,
PHILADELPHIA, PENNSYLVANIA

Anyone who might be giving your child anything at all to eat needs to know how to read food labels and look for ingredients that could be a problem. For people with a true food allergy, even a microscopic amount of the food is enough to trigger a reaction. To a child allergic to peanuts, cutting a bologna sandwich with the same knife you just used to spread peanut butter could be deadly.

Children who have life-threatening allergic reactions to foods, called anaphylactic reactions, should carry an epinephrine auto-injector (Epi-pen) with them everywhere they go. Epinephrine can stop the allergic reaction and open the child's airways in the event of an emergency. Anyone caring for the child should know how to use the Epi-pen.

Many people who think they have a food allergy, however, actually have a food "intolerance," according to Dr. Feldman. People who just have a food intolerance can generally eat small amounts of the food in question without experiencing symptoms, and their symptoms usually are not life-threatening.

PET ALLERGIES

If your child has an allergy to pet dander, whether or not you need to say good-bye to your pet depends on how bad your child's symptoms are. If the symptoms aren't severe, you can do other things to limit your child's exposure to pet dander.

If your child is allergic but you are keeping your pet, do away with as much upholstered furniture and carpeting as possible in your home. Even if you never allow the pet into the room, animal dander can be brought in on people's clothing and shoes, and stick to upholstery and carpeting.

—STUART ABRAMSON, M.D., PH.D.,
TEXAS CHILDREN'S HOSPITAL

Create off-limit areas for the pet—especially your child's bedroom—so that you can keep these rooms extra clean and free of pet dander. And bathe your pet frequently to help reduce the amount of dander the pet sheds. Even cats can learn to tolerate baths if you start working with them as kittens, doctors say.

After you get rid of a cat, it takes six months for the level of allergens in the house to go down, so don't be surprised if your child's symptoms don't improve right away. Cat allergen is in the saliva, which gets on the fur when the cat bathes itself, and is then shed throughout the house.

—ROBERT FELDMAN, M.D.,
CHILDREN'S HOSPITAL OF NEW YORK

If your child is going to visit someone who has a pet, make sure the pet is out of the room during the visit, and have your child avoid sitting on the carpet or upholstered furniture, where animal dander is most likely to cling. Also remind your child not to rub her eyes or face, and to wash her hands carefully after the visit. Dander rubbed in the nose or eyes—even if very little is present—can cause an allergic reaction.

—STUART ABRAMSON, M.D., PH.D.,
TEXAS CHILDREN'S HOSPITAL

You might also consider letting your child have some other type of pet. Lizards and reptiles are free of dander, though you'll need to make sure your child washes carefully after touching or feeding the pet or cleaning its cage to protect against Salmonella infection. Fish are a safe bet. Your child might even be able to have a small cage pet such as a hamster, rat, or Guinea pig. Some breeds of cats and dogs are known to be less allergenic; ask your vet for recommendations.

Because an allergist cannot test for sensitivity to a type of pet the child has never been exposed to, consider first borrowing the school hamster for a few days, or having your child visit a friend who has a hamster frequently over a period of a few weeks. This will give your child enough exposure that you can tell whether the hamster will be a problem before you bring one home and let your child get attached to it.

—ANDREA McCOY,
TEMPLE UNIVERSITY CHILDREN'S MEDICAL CENTER,
PHILADELPHIA, PENNSYLVANIA

WHEN TO CALL THE DOCTOR

If you find yourself giving your child over-the-counter antihistamines on a regular basis, or otherwise suspect your child has allergies, it's a good idea to contact your doctor for an evaluation. Doctors can help you learn to minimize the amount of allergens in your child's environment and prescribe nondrowsy medications that will relieve your child's symptoms. If your child has severe allergic reactions, your child's doctor will prescribe an Epi-pen, which could save her life.

If your child has a serious allergic reaction, seek emergency medical attention.

Signs of life-threatening allergic reaction:

- Difficulty breathing
- Wheezing
- Persistent cough
- Change in voice
- Pain in the throat
- Swelling inside the mouth
- Fainting
- Light-headedness
- Sudden vomiting or diarrhea

Hives that spread all over the body can look scary, but aren't as dangerous as a reaction involving the airway. However, you should still seek medical attention for serious cases of hives, because your child's next reaction might be more severe.

Anemia

About 20 percent of children in the United States will be anemic at some point before they reach age eighteen—most likely during the first year of life or adolescence. These are times of high growth and potentially poor diet, which can make it difficult for the body to get the iron needed to make red blood cells. Premature babies are also at severe risk, as they don't stay in the womb long enough to acquire the complete supply of iron from their mothers. Other causes include:

- Conditions like sickle cell anemia or some forms of cancer, which inhibit red blood cell production
- Conditions such as hemolysis or sickle cell, which destroy red blood cells in the body

- When blood cells are lost through internal or external bleeding—even heavy menstrual bleeding

Anemia, especially in children, can be hard to spot. All the symptoms tend to be written off as "just part of childhood." In babies and small children, the most common symptoms are irritability, fatigue, and paleness. Toddlers who are iron-deficient may try eating dirt or chewing on inedible objects. In school-age children, you might notice behavior problems and a lack of interest in school. The only way to know for certain whether your child is anemic is to have his blood tested.

Quick test for anemia:

- Fan back your child's fingers gently and look at the creases in the hand. They should be red.
- Examine your child's lips. They should be pink.
- Put a finger under your child's eye and pull the bottom lid down gently. The undersurface of the lid should be pink.

If this is not the case, you should have your child tested for anemia.

—GREGORY A. YANIK, M.D., C.S.,
MOTT CHILDREN'S HOSPITAL
AT THE UNIVERSITY OF MICHIGAN

Anemia may be hard to spot, but it isn't harmless. The heart has to work harder to make up for the shortage of blood cells, and over the long term the condition can impact a child's growth, cause developmental problems, and even lead to an enlarged heart or heart failure.

Doctors agree that all children should be tested for anemia by age one, and again during adolescence.

FIRST RESPONSE

GETTING A DIAGNOSIS

If your child has been diagnosed as anemic, it's important to find out why. Treatment for the forms of anemia can differ, and the iron supplements used to treat iron-deficiency anemia could be harmful to children with other forms of anemia. A doctor's care is essential.

If the cause of your child's anemia is iron deficiency, you should also ask whether your child is at risk for lead poisoning. The mechanism that allows the body to absorb the necessary iron also allows it to absorb toxic lead. When the body is iron-deficient, this mechanism naturally speeds up and makes the body more susceptible to taking in lead.

> If your child is diagnosed as iron-deficient and you are in a situation where she is at risk for lead exposure (e.g., you live in an older house), ask your doctor about giving your child a lead test.
> —JIM KORB, M.D.,
> MATTEL CHILDREN'S HOSPITAL AT UCLA

If your doctor diagnoses iron-deficiency anemia, she will most likely prescribe iron supplements and perhaps some dietary changes for your child. Other forms of anemia, such as sickle cell and hemolysis, are treated in other ways.

COMFORT CARE

If your child has anemia with symptoms, he'll need a good dose of TLC. If the anemia is due to iron deficiency, you'll have to help make taking the iron supplements easier, and perhaps even manage some dietary changes for your family.

Resources: Cause and Effect

Cooley's Anemia Foundation
129-09 26th Avenue
Flushing, NY 11354
(718) 321-2873
www.cooleysanemia.org

**Sickle Cell Disease
Association of America**
200 Corporate Point,
Suite 495
Culver City, CA 90230-8727
www.sicklecelldisease.org
(800) 421-8453

**Aplastic Anemia Foundation of
America**
P.O. Box 613
Annapolis, MD 21404
(800) 747-2820
www.aplastic.org

Sickle Cell Information Center
P.O. Box 109
Grady Memorial Hospital

80 Butler Street
Atlanta, GA 30335
(404) 616-3572
www.emory.edu/PEDS/
SICKLE

Fanconi Anemia Research Fund
1902 Jefferson Street,
Suite 2
Eugene, OR 97405
(541) 687-4658
www.fanconi.org

Diamond Blackfan Registry
Attn: Adrianna Vlachos, M.D.
Schneider Children's
Hospital
269-01 76th Avenue
New Hyde Park, NY 11040
(718) 470-3460

SYMPTOMS

Fatigue, behavior problems, and poor performance in school can all be the result of anemia. If your child is dealing with these symptoms—especially as they relate to school—it may be helpful to talk with her teacher. Explain the problem and what is being done to correct it, then come up with a plan for making up missed assignments or doing some type of extra-credit work once your child is feeling better. But don't forget to allow time for your child to recover.

Behavior problems can be a bit trickier to deal with, particularly with toddlers, who can't understand why they feel so tired and cranky. An explanation to your child's teacher is still in order, but it may not excuse your child from the consequences. Do your best to work things out, and keep in mind that your child's attitude—at least in regard to his anemia—should begin to improve with a couple of weeks of treatment.

In the meantime, make sure you follow your doctor's advice, and that your child is eating right and getting plenty of rest.

SUFFERING THROUGH SUPPLEMENTS

If your child's anemia is caused by iron deficiency, the only way to correct it is with a prescription iron supplement. The amount of iron found in over-the-counter supplements isn't enough to replenish the body's supply, and higher doses should be given only under a doctor's supervision. *Iron overdoses can be fatal* and are the number one cause of poisoning deaths in children. If you have any type of iron supplement in the house, keep it well out of reach of children.

Supplements can usually clear up a case of iron-deficiency anemia in around three months. Unfortunately, the cure does not come without side effects.

Constipation

The most common complaint associated with iron supplements is constipation. While it's not usually a problem for people taking a simple multivitamin with iron, children on high-dose iron supplements can be affected.

In mild cases, simple dietary adjustments may solve the problem.

Make sure your child takes in lots of fiber and not too much milk. Cereals are the best way to get fiber into kids.
—ROBERT HAYASHI, M.D.,
ST. LOUIS CHILDREN'S HOSPITAL

Lots of extra water, juice, and other fluids can help relieve your child's constipation. Whole-grain breads are also good sources of fiber, as are dried fruits. You can even sneak a little wheat germ into soups and sauces.

Some doctors think over-the-counter medications may also be worth a try.

A stool softener, such as Docusate, can be taken daily to help with constipation.
—NATHAN HAGSTROM, M.D.,
CONNECTICUT CHILDREN'S MEDICAL CENTER

Be careful to choose something specifically made for children. Harsh laxatives are not recommended and could cause painful cramping. If the constipation is severe, consult your pediatrician.

Ask your doctor about giving your child a lower daily dose of iron and correcting the problem over a longer period of time. Taking less iron may help relieve constipation.
—JIM KORB, M.D.,
MATTEL CHILDREN'S HOSPITAL AT UCLA

Upset Stomach

Iron in doses high enough to treat anemia can also upset a child's stomach. This is especially true since iron is usually given on an empty stomach, to help absorb as much as possible into the bloodstream.

If stomach upset is problematic, talk to your doctor
about giving the iron in divided doses two or three
times a day. Occasionally, a physician will need to
decrease the total dose of prescribed iron due to stomach upset.

> —JENNIFER MAYER, M.D.,
> ALL CHILDREN'S HOSPITAL,
> ST. PETERSBURG, FLORIDA

If this doesn't work, you may want to try giving the supplement with food, though the prescription may tell you not
to. Certain foods—namely those containing vitamin C—can
actually help the body absorb more iron. Doctors recommend you avoid tea, bran, and milk, since they can keep the
iron from being absorbed properly.

Make sure there is a thirty- to sixty-minute gap between
drinking milk and taking iron.

> —MICHAEL RECHT, M.D.,
> PHOENIX CHILDREN'S HOSPITAL

Give supplements to babies straight from the dropper.
Do not mix the supplement in a bottle of milk or formula. For young children, it's best to use either the
elixir or syrup form of iron supplement. These are palatable, and you don't have to use much.

> —HOWARD PEARSON, M.D.,
> YALE–NEW HAVEN CHILDREN'S HOSPITAL

Diarrhea

A much less common but equally troubling complaint associated with iron supplements is diarrhea. This is usually cor-
rectable with a slight change in diet. The BRAT diet (bananas,
rice, applesauce, and toast) is commonly recommended by
doctors because it's gentle on the digestive system.

If your child develops diarrhea, give the supplement with foods like bananas. Avoid giving it with fruit or juice, or other foods that might be contributing.

—MICHAEL RECHT, M.D.,
PHOENIX CHILDREN'S HOSPITAL

Again, if the medication is causing severe symptoms, call your doctor and explain the situation. She may be able to decrease the dosage or change the prescription slightly.

Stained Teeth

Iron supplements for children usually come in a liquid form, which can cause some staining of the teeth. Make sure your child has something to drink after taking the supplement.

Have your child take his liquid iron from the dropper that comes in the medicine bottle, or through a straw. This prevents contact with the teeth and staining.

—JILL REEL, M.D., AND PATRICK STEINAUER, M.D.,
BOYS TOWN NATIONAL RESEARCH HOSPITAL,
OMAHA, NEBRASKA

Have your child wash down iron supplements with fruit juices or water to help prevent staining of the teeth.

—BETSY SONNENBLICK, R.N., M.S.N., C.P.N.P.,
ST. JOSEPH'S CHILDREN'S HOSPITAL, NEW JERSEY

After taking iron supplements, have your child brush his teeth with a baking soda toothpaste.

—JIM KORB, M.D.,
MATTEL CHILDREN'S HOSPITAL AT UCLA

If your child's teeth still show some staining, don't worry. Doctors agree that the condition is temporary and should fade a few weeks after your child finishes the round of supplements.

The supplement will likely change the color of your child's stool, turning it much darker than usual. This is normal and does not indicate a health problem.

CHANGING THE DIET

If your child is iron-deficient, your pediatrician will probably recommend some changes in her diet, both during treatment and as a follow-up preventive measure. Doctors agree that eating a wide variety of healthy foods is the best way to take in enough iron.

> If you have to change your child's diet to include more iron, these changes should be made for the whole family. This will make them easier for the child to accept, and help your whole family eat healthier.
>
> —JIM KORB, M.D.,
> MATTEL CHILDREN'S HOSPITAL AT UCLA

Spinach and Beyond

It is important to note that, no matter what you may have heard about Popeye's favorite canned cuisine, the best sources of iron tend to be meats, not spinach. This is because 40 to 50 percent of the iron in meat is absorbed by the body, compared to only 10 percent of that in vegetables.

IRON: RECOMMENDED DAILY ALLOWANCE

0 to 6 months: 6 mg
7 to 12 months: 10 mg
1 to 10 years: 10 mg
Adolescent boys: 12 mg
Adolescent girls: 15 mg

For Babies

The American Academy of Pediatrics recommends that all babies receive breast milk for at least the first six months of life. And doctors agree that while breast milk is relatively low in iron, the iron that is there is absorbed very efficiently by the baby. Babies also begin life with a good supply of iron passed on from their mothers during pregnancy.

> The store of iron a baby builds up in the womb begins to be depleted at about six months of age. If you are breast-feeding, this is a good time to begin an iron supplement. If you are using formula, it should be iron-fortified, in which case a supplement is not necessary.
> —MICHAEL RECHT, M.D.,
> PHOENIX CHILDREN'S HOSPITAL

Parents who use formula often worry that iron-fortified formulas will cause digestive problems for their babies, in much the way that a high-dose iron supplement might. But doctors agree this isn't the case. Studies have shown no difference in digestion between babies taking iron-fortified formula and those on the low-iron variety. Any difficulties are more likely the result of some other ingredient in the formula. If your baby is having trouble with high-iron formula, try switching brands rather than moving to a low-iron version.

> Fortified cereals are an excellent way to get iron into the diet, and you can use fortified rice-cereal powder as a thickening agent in other pureed baby foods, which tend to be watery. This adds an extra amount of iron. Meats should be introduced at six to eight months if your child will accept them.
> —JIM KORB, M.D.,
> MATTEL CHILDREN'S HOSPITAL AT UCLA

In addition, doctors recommend that all babies begin eating iron-rich foods at six months of age. Children who aren't introduced to solid foods at this time tend to have much lower iron stores in the body.

One mistake many parents make is switching children from breast milk or formula to cow's milk before their baby is a year old. Unlike breast milk and formula, which both provide iron and a variety of other nutrients, cow's milk is low in iron and shouldn't take the place of iron-rich foods.

In addition, cow's milk can create digestive problems for babies. It often causes irritation in the lining of the intestines, which can cause mild internal bleeding that brings on or contributes to anemia.

Toddlers

Even after your child enters toddlerhood, when cow's milk is more easily handled by the digestive system, too much milk can cause problems in the diet and contribute to iron deficiency.

> We recommend a minimum of sixteen ounces a day (for calcium, protein, and vitamin D) and a maximum of twenty-four ounces a day (the point where it begins to affect the rest of the child's diet).
> —KATHY MCGEORGE, M.D.,
> CHILDREN'S HOSPITAL OF MICHIGAN

Again, don't treat cow's milk as if it were breast milk or formula. Mother's milk and formula are both designed to be a balanced meal for the child, while cow's milk is designed to be a balanced meal for a baby cow.

> If you are just switching your one-year-old from formula or breast milk to cow's milk, make sure you add enough

iron-rich foods to the diet to compensate for the loss of
iron from the formula/breast milk.

—JOHN M. OLSSON, M.D.,
ST. JOSEPH'S CHILDREN'S HOSPITAL, NEW JERSEY

You may find this more difficult than it sounds. Toddlers
can be picky eaters, and putting together a balanced diet for a
tiny tummy may seem like a Herculean task. Doctors advise
that you just continue to offer them as many types of iron-
rich foods as they will eat. And remember, your toddler does
not need to eat nearly as much as you do to collect a full day's
supply of nutrients.

Most people forget how little toddlers really need to eat.
A serving of meat for a one-year-old can be as little as
one tablespoon. Just offer your toddler a serving of meat
once a day, and make sure he or she eats fortified
breads and cereals and peanut butter.

—JIM KORB, M.D.,
MATTEL CHILDREN'S HOSPITAL AT UCLA

Older Children

As picky as toddlers are, they may be easier to convince into a
healthy diet than your older child—especially an adolescent.
Remember that adolescence is another high-risk time for
iron-deficiency anemia, and it's still up to you to help your
teen get adequate iron. Doctors stress the importance of setting a good example with your own eating habits. But if
you're locked into other battles with your teen, the food
battle may best be left to someone else.

If you have trouble convincing your child of the importance of a good diet, have either their doctor or a

dietitian talk with them, or maybe some other third
party they trust.

—Michael Recht, M.D.,
Phoenix Children's Hospital

Taking a bit of extra care with the food your child eats
can help add iron. A few simple changes in what you put into
the grocery cart can make a big difference.

Iron-Rich Foods

Food	Serving size	Iron (mg)
Breakfast cereals	¾ to 1 cup	Check the label
Raisins	¼ cup	1.0
Enriched breads (white)	2 slices	1.4
Enriched breads (wheat)	2 slices	1.7
Enriched pasta	1 cup	1.9
Baked beans (canned)	½ cup	2.0
Lean ground beef	3 oz.	3.9
Pork chop	3 oz.	3.5
Tuna, canned	3.5 oz.	1.0
Chicken breast	3 oz.	0.9
Chicken thigh	2.3 oz.	1.2
Prune juice	½ cup	1.5
Spinach, cooked	½ cup	2.0
Broccoli, cooked	½ cup	0.6
Rice, white enriched	1 cup	1.8
Peas, frozen	½ cup	1.3
Salmon, canned	3 oz.	0.7
Potato	1 medium	0.62
Peanut butter	2 tablespoons	0.62
Egg	1 large	0.72

Watch the labels on your child's breakfast cereal to make sure they have an adequate amount of fortified iron. Many kids' cereals are very low. If you're planning on this as a major source of iron in your child's diet, then a serving should contain 25 percent or more of the RDA of iron.

—JOHN M. OLSSON, M.D.,
ST. JOSEPH'S CHILDREN'S HOSPITAL, NEW JERSEY

Keep iron-rich foods and snacks readily available. Balance your child's diet over time. Don't focus too much on day-to-day eating.

—DANNY WOOD, M.D.,
THE CHILDREN'S HOSPITAL OF SOUTHWEST FLORIDA

The way you and your family approach the cooking of meals can also make a difference. A child who is involved in choosing and preparing the family meals will be more likely to pay attention to what she eats, and to follow your suggestions.

Cook in cast-iron pots as much as possible, as this adds iron to the food you are preparing. Serve orange or grapefruit juice with meals, so the vitamin C they contain will help maximize the iron in the food.

—JENNIFER MAYER, M.D.,
ALL CHILDREN'S HOSPITAL,
ST. PETERSBURG, FLORIDA

Try making baked-potato wedges instead of french fries. Potato peels are a good source of iron, and if you make them yourself, you can leave the peel on and sneak a little extra iron into your child's meal.

—JOHN M. OLSSON, M.D.,
ST. JOSEPH'S CHILDREN'S HOSPITAL, NEW JERSEY

Watching an adolescent's diet can be especially tough if the family has a hectic schedule and doesn't often sit down at the table together for meals. Doctors agree that one of the best ways to improve kids' eating habits is to institute regular sit-down meals as much as possible.

In addition, don't base your assessment of a child's diet on any particular day. Everyone has good eating days and bad eating days. The best plan of attack is to try to balance your child's nutrition over a week or so.

OVER-THE-COUNTER SUPPLEMENTS

Parents may wonder whether they should give their child some sort of over-the-counter vitamin supplement to help make up for bad eating days. There's no consensus from doctors about this. Some recommend them for most or all children; some think they're a good idea during the infant years and adolescence, when a child is most at risk for iron deficiency. Others think children should never be given vitamin supplements except under a doctor's care.

All doctors seem to agree that the best way for the body to take in nutrients is through a balanced and healthy diet. And most concede that an over-the-counter multivitamin supplement with iron certainly would do no harm, as long as the vitamins are taken as directed and kept out of the reach of children.

> Stay away from "natural" supplements, because they are not tested for contaminants. A contaminant or bacteria that is harmless to an adult could prove disastrous for a baby's developing immune system.
>
> —MICHAEL RECHT, M.D.,
> PHOENIX CHILDREN'S HOSPITAL

Doctors do recommend supplements for premature babies, who are especially at risk. These, however, should be given on the advice of your pediatrician. As always, if you are concerned about your child's eating habits and aren't sure whether you want to give a supplement, ask your doctor's advice. He can perform the necessary tests to let you know whether a supplement is truly needed, and can give you his views on whether or not they're helpful.

WHEN TO CALL THE DOCTOR

Your child's doctor will likely want to follow up in about three months. However, if your child is taking an iron supplement and having severe side effects, call the doctor immediately. You should also call if any symptoms your child is experiencing haven't begun to improve within two or three weeks of starting treatment.

Even if your child's symptoms do improve, be sure to keep your scheduled follow-up appointment. The symptoms are likely to go away long before the proper amount of iron has been restored to your child's body. The only way to tell for sure if the anemia has been corrected is to have a follow-up blood test.

If your child is still iron-deficient after the full course of treatment, or has had a relapse, the doctor should begin looking for other causes for the condition beyond poor dietary intake.

Asthma

Asthma is the most common chronic childhood illness. Close to five million children in the United States have asthma, according to the American Academy of Allergy, Asthma & Immunology. Since the 1980s, the number of children under five with the disease has jumped at least 160 percent, so an increasing number of families are learning to cope with the condition. The consequences can be serious. Asthma is now the number one reason for childhood hospitalizations in the United States.

The condition affects the breathing tubes in the lungs and, when triggered, causes swelling that makes them too narrow to let air in and out comfortably. When a child with asthma is exposed to something that "triggers" it (e.g., dog hair, pollen, having a cold), his breathing tubes swell. The child may then begin to cough, wheeze, and have trouble breathing. This is an asthma attack.

Doctors report that a large number of patients begin to "outgrow" their asthma, or at least to see a reduction in their symptoms and the number of asthma attacks, as they become teenagers.

FIRST RESPONSE

COPING WITH ASTHMA ATTACKS

Note: If this is your child's first asthma attack, call the doctor immediately.

Signs of Mild Asthma Attack
• Mild difficulty breathing
• Breathing slightly faster than normal
• Mild wheezing, cough, shortness of breath, or chest tightness
• Peak flow rate of 70 to 90 percent of child's personal best

Signs of Moderate Asthma Attack
• Moderate difficulty breathing
• Breathing moderately faster than normal
• Child is unable to finish a whole sentence without stopping to take a breath
• Moderate wheezing, cough, shortness of breath, or chest tightness
• Skin might appear pale
• Slight to moderate "drawing in" of the muscles between the ribs when the child breathes

- Peak flow rate of 50 to 70 percent of the child's personal best

Signs of Severe Asthma Attack
- Extreme difficulty breathing
- Breathing much faster than normal, or much slower and labored
- Inability to finish a whole sentence without stopping for a breath
- Severe wheezing, cough, shortness of breath, or chest tightness
- Poor skin color
- Severe "drawing in" of the muscles in the neck, abdomen, and chest when the child breathes
- Drowsiness
- Peak flow rate less than 50 percent of the child's personal best

If your child has asthma, work out and write down an asthma attack plan with your child's doctors, and keep it in a place where it is easy to find—even at three A.M. This will help you stay calm and make sure nothing is forgotten.

Remove your child from the environment that may have triggered the attack. If the child is allergic to cats and there is a cat present, move away from the cat. [Don't just remove the cat; this will leave behind some fur or dander, which are triggers.] If the environment is moldy, musty, or dusty, move to a cleaner, drier place. Look for a quiet place with good air circulation.

—Nikki Nair, M.D.,
Boys Town National Research Hospital,
Omaha, Nebraska

The next step when your child is having an attack is to evaluate its severity, then follow the plan for that situation.

Be sure to keep your child's asthma medications close at hand, and check periodically to see that none have expired. Give medications as dictated by the plan, and remember that it is better to give them too soon than too late.

> If your house was on fire, you wouldn't throw "just a little" water on it and wait to see what happens. So don't do this with your child's asthma. Give the full recommended dose of medication to prevent attacks and to keep them from getting worse.
>
> —STEVEN KANENGISER, M.D., F.A.A.P., F.C.C.P.,
> ST. JOSEPH'S MEDICAL CENTER,
> PATERSON, NEW JERSEY

Stay calm, and help your child stay calm. This will make the attack less stressful. Don't make light of your child's reactions to the attack, but don't panic. If you do, she may hide future symptoms or attacks for fear of upsetting *you*.

> Read your child a favorite story, watch a favorite video together, or play some music he likes. Doing anything your child finds soothing will help.
>
> —RON FERDMAN, M.D.,
> CHILDRENS HOSPITAL LOS ANGELES

Don't delay giving medication in favor of calming tactics. Remember, it's the inability to breathe that is frightening your child. The sooner his medication begins to work and he can breathe, the sooner he'll begin to calm down.

While the medication is working, keep your child as comfortable as possible.

Don't make your child lie down. Children having an asthma attack usually feel better sitting up, as this helps them to feel in control. Giving your child room-temperature water to drink may also help him feel better.

—MARY PAT HEMSTREET, M.D.,
BIRMINGHAM CHILDREN'S HOSPITAL

Try giving a cup of warm tea or broth, relaxing your child in a bath (after giving medication), or gently rubbing her back.

—LESLIE D. QUINN,
ST. JOSEPH'S CHILDREN'S HOSPITAL, NEW JERSEY

Cold air can be a trigger for asthma, so make sure your child stays in a warm room if she's having an asthma attack. Humidity also aggravates asthma, so avoid putting a humidifier in your child's room.

—GABRIEL HADDAD, M.D.,
YALE–NEW HAVEN CHILDREN'S HOSPITAL

If the medication doesn't appear to be working, call your doctor or go to the hospital as your asthma plan dictates.

After the attack is over, sit down and do your best to figure out what triggered it, how everyone reacted, and what you might be able to do differently next time. Share this information with your child's doctor, either in a follow-up phone call or at your next office visit.

COMFORT CARE

You will have more than just your child's "acute" episodes to deal with. Asthma is a chronic condition which, in most children, requires ongoing care. Learning about and monitoring your child's asthma, preventive medication, and the proper attitude can help him keep the disease in check and lead a normal life.

TRIGGERS

You should know what triggers your child's asthma: anything from playing in a soccer game to dust, pollen, or pet hair. Knowing the triggers means you can help your child avoid them (not letting her play with her friend's new puppy or kitten) or help prepare for them (giving medication before the big soccer match).

If you have a pet in the house that absolutely cannot be given up, you can still reduce its impact on your child's asthma. Doctors recommend keeping the pet outdoors if at all possible, but at the very least, keep it out of the child's bedroom. Since your child spends roughly one-third of his or her time there, it is the most important place to keep trigger-free. You can also help by removing carpets and upholstered furniture, which harbor pet dander, from the home, and by using a vacuum cleaner with a HEPA filter to clean up as much dander as possible.

You can find out which triggers apply to your own child only through careful observation.

Keep a diary about your child's asthma. Write down when symptoms occur and what's going on when they occur. This can provide valuable information for your child's doctor and help you determine what triggers his asthma.
—MARC S. MCMORRIS, M.D.,
UNIVERSITY OF MICHIGAN CHILDREN'S HOSPITAL

Does your child cough whenever you vacuum the house? Dust mites are probably one of her triggers. Does he start to wheeze whenever he pets the neighbor's cat? Pet dander likely aggravates his asthma. Does she have trouble breathing when she goes down into the basement? The culprit is probably the mold in the air.

> Consider having your child evaluated by an allergy specialist. She can help you identify triggers and even plan preventive measures.
> —NIKKI NAIR, M.D.,
>   BOYS TOWN NATIONAL RESEARCH HOSPITAL,
>   OMAHA, NEBRASKA

Don't be frustrated if you can't pinpoint all of your child's triggers right away. Doctors report that asthma changes with the seasons, and also as your child grows. Understanding and dealing with it is an ongoing process.

Pulling the Trigger

Knowing what triggers your child's asthma is essential for both of you. You can eliminate or control some triggers so that they don't bother your child. Others you can prepare for, preventing attacks or making the ones that do happen less severe and less frequent.

- Upper respiratory infections, such as colds, are the most common asthma triggers. If your child has asthma attacks with every cold, work to control the symptoms quickly to help prevent an attack.
- Exercise is another very common trigger. No one wants to keep a child from running and playing, or from participating in her favorite sport, and it is very rare that a child's asthma is so extreme that sports must be eliminated completely. Giving your child a puff from the inhaler just before the big game, and

keeping medication on hand during games and
practice, may be all you need to do to keep your child
on the field.

- Humidity and mold are especially prevalent with
changes in the weather. Buy a humidity gauge and
keep the level in your home between 30 and 50
percent to minimize mold growth. Venting bathrooms
and finished basements is essential.

- Allergens such as dust mites, pollen, animal dander,
and smoke can be controlled with some work on your
part. Fish or lizards are preferred pets for children
bothered by animal hair. If you must have a dog or
cat, don't allow it in your child's bedroom. Close the
windows and run the air conditioner to help with
pollen; damp mopping and vacuuming with a HEPA
(High Efficiency Particle Arresting) filter, can deal
with the dust. HEPA vacuums are designed to catch
even the smallest particles, such as pet dander and
mold spores. And, of course, don't smoke.

- Irritants like fumes from cleaners, perfumes, paint,
and kerosene lamps and heaters can trigger attacks.
If you must paint or use cleaners with strong fumes,
make sure you do it while your child is out of the
house. And save the perfume or cologne for times
when you won't be hugging your child.

Exercise environmental control. Get rid of smoking and
pets in your home if these are your child's triggers.
Keep windows closed to control mold and pollen.

—ROBERT STRUNK, M.D.,
ST. LOUIS CHILDREN'S HOSPITAL

You should also be aware of the early signs that your
child is headed for an asthma attack. Contrary to popular
belief, most asthma attacks do not come on in an instant.

They build gradually to the point where the child cannot breathe.

> Listen to your child, because kids know what's going on with their bodies. Sometimes a child can recognize a symptom that isn't apparent to anyone else but is a precursor to every attack they have. This can serve as an early-warning mechanism, so that parents can give medication soon enough to fend off the attack.
> —MARY ANN LEWIS, DR.P.H., R.N., F.A.A.N.,
> MATTEL CHILDREN'S HOSPITAL AT UCLA

This warning signal could be anything from a slight cough or tickling in the throat, to a fit of sneezing, to a mild shortness of breath or funny feeling in the chest. Whatever it may be, if your child is old enough to tell you that this is a signal of an impending attack, take it seriously and give the appropriate medication.

MEDICATION

Most children who have asthma are on some sort of daily preventive medication.

One of the disadvantages of asthma medication is that it often requires the use of an inhaler—a small canister that sprays a mist of medication to be breathed into the lungs—or a nebulizer, a machine that compresses medication into a mist. Learn how to use these devices from your child's doctor, or through one of the many asthma support groups that offer family education classes. Then be prepared to help and coach your child on a day-to-day basis.

> Don't give instructions about proper medication technique in the middle of a crisis. You will have more success if you do your teaching when your child is calm and

not having an asthma attack. Ideally, children should learn in groups, since they can learn techniques most easily from other children.

—MARY ANN LEWIS, DR.P.H., R.N., F.A.A.N.,
MATTEL CHILDREN'S HOSPITAL AT UCLA

Even after your child reaches a point where she can take the medication without your help, you will need to make sure she doesn't forget or slide into improper techniques.

Ask your child's doctor to watch her use her medication and provide refresher instruction at every visit. This will help ensure that your child continues to use the medication correctly.

—MARY PAT HEMSTREET, M.D.,
BIRMINGHAM CHILDREN'S HOSPITAL

Of course, the best technique in the world won't help if you and your child forget the medication completely. Remembering may be especially difficult when your child is doing well, but adhering to a schedule is essential to keeping your child's asthma under control. Your doctor may be able to choose a medication your child doesn't have to take more than twice a day, or morning and night, which will be less of a hassle.

Find a time to give the drug that the child can remember, and link it to something else they do twice a day. If that activity is brushing their teeth, then put the medication next to the toothbrush. If they switch on the TV every morning and right after school, store it on top of the TV. If they go straight to the refrigerator for breakfast, and for a snack after school, keep the medication on the fridge.

—RICK VINUYA, M.D.,
CHILDREN'S HOSPITAL OF MICHIGAN

You can also make medication less of a hassle by requesting the simplest form available. An inhaler takes only two or three minutes to deliver the medication, while a nebulizer takes up to thirty (although concentrated forms of medication can cut this to fifteen). Some medications come in once-a-day pill form. Ask your doctor if a quicker and simpler medication would work for your child.

Taste is one factor that can cause asthma patients of any age to complain. Here's another key area where your child can have a choice. There is generally more than one effective medication, and since each tastes different, you can let your child choose the one he prefers.

> Even if he doesn't care for any of the medications he tries, a child may be more willing to take a medication he has chosen himself. Rinsing the mouth out with water—or even juice or milk—may help mask the taste, as will brushing the teeth immediately after using the medication. Using a spacer [see p. 49] also helps minimize the bad taste, since the heavier particles fall into the spacer and not into the mouth.
>
> —RON FERDMAN, M.D.,
> CHILDRENS HOSPITAL LOS ANGELES

If your child's medication is available this way, a dry powder inhaler (DPI) might be preferable. This type of inhaler has no bad-tasting propellant. Your child simply dispenses the appropriate amount of powder and inhales it.

Failing to use preventive medications can even lead to overuse of "rescue" medications, which can increase the side effects associated with these medications. Don't let your child stop taking her medication without first talking to your doctor, but do make sure she is evaluated periodically for correct dosages. If a child is doing well, the doctor may reduce the dosages.

Babies and Toddlers

Your biggest challenge if your child is under age two or three is probably getting him to sit still to take his medication. Fight the good fight and don't give up. This medication is the key to controlling your child's asthma.

> When giving medication to babies and toddlers, give them choices in matters where they can have a choice. Let them shake the inhaler themselves. Let them choose where they will sit to have their nebulizer treatment. But be completely inflexible when it comes to actually *giving* the medication. Once your child has learned that she *will* get her medication every time you say she will, she may give up fighting you. Getting into a routine—much as you do at bedtime—may also help your child be more accepting of the medicine.
>
> —RON FERDMAN, M.D.,
> CHILDRENS HOSPITAL LOS ANGELES

Help your child make the connection that this medication eases her breathing. Once she realizes this, she will almost certainly fight the inhaler or nebulizer less.

> When introducing your baby or toddler to an inhaler and spacer, let him spend some time playing with the device so that he won't be afraid of it when the time comes to use it.
>
> —GABRIEL HADDAD, M.D.,
> YALE–NEW HAVEN CHILDREN'S HOSPITAL

If your baby is using an inhaler, he should also be using a spacer. This device—available either as a rigid plastic tube or a collapsible plastic bag—gets more medication into the lungs and leaves less in the mouth. The inhaler fires the medication into the spacer, where it can be mixed with air and inhaled slowly and more easily. Of the two types of spacers, doctors recommend the noncollapsible one for babies.

> A paper or Styrofoam cup makes a good homemade spacer for babies who aren't comfortable with the face mask.
> —LESLIE D. QUINN, M.D.,
> ST. JOSEPH'S CHILDREN'S HOSPITAL, NEW JERSEY

Your baby may also need a nebulizer. This means she'll have to sit quietly near a loud machine while you hold a plastic mask over her nose and mouth—a challenge, to say the least.

> Let the baby get used to the nebulizer mask with the machine turned off—before it's necessary to give a treatment. This should be done at a time when both you and the baby are calm and relaxed.
> —ROBERT STRUNK, M.D.,
> ST. LOUIS CHILDREN'S HOSPITAL

> Don't give the treatment while the baby is asleep. If he wakes during the treatment, he'll be more frightened than ever and may develop a fear of going to sleep. And even if you're successful, failing to address your child's fear now may only make it more difficult in the future. Instead, try giving the treatment along with some pleasant experience like watching a favorite video or reading a story. This may make it more palatable.
> —RON FERDMAN, M.D.,
> CHILDRENS HOSPITAL LOS ANGELES

You can make the nebulizer mask less frightening by bringing a little fun into the treatment.

Decorate the nebulizer and mask. Glue ears on it or
draw bunny whiskers. Adapt a fairy tale so that the hero
or heroine has asthma, then work the nebulizer into the
story and tell the story during nebulizer treatments. You
can even decorate Styrofoam cups and substitute them
for the face mask to add more variety.

—RICK VINUYA, M.D.,
CHILDREN'S HOSPITAL OF MICHIGAN

Even if you don't decorate it, a plain drinking cup will
likely be less frightening to a baby or toddler than the nebulizer mask. Some children are also afraid of the noise the
nebulizer makes. Quieter models are available, but these tend
to be expensive. Playing music, perhaps with headphones,
or a favorite video may help drown out the sound of the
machine.

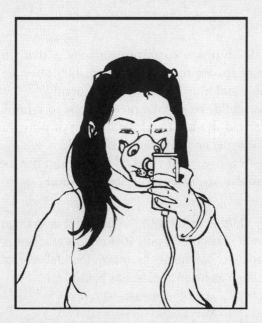

Decorating a nebulizer mask as a puppet for a frightened child.

School-age Children

When she's five or six, you can explain to your child why the medication is so important. Giving choices begins to be more important at this age, as does teaching your child to use her medications on her own.

> Consider letting your school-age child trade her spacer's or nebulizer's face mask for a mouthpiece, which will make her feel more in control. This is also a good time to trade the rigid clear plastic spacer for an "inspirease bag," a clear plastic bag that collapses and inflates with the child's breath. These let the child see if she's inhaling the medications correctly, and let parents see if she is inhaling the full dose (since the entire bag must be deflated for the child to get the whole dose).
>
> —Ron Ferdman, M.D.,
> Childrens Hospital Los Angeles

One disadvantage to inspirease bags is that, unlike the rigid type of spacer, they are not washable. They are also not very durable and must be replaced frequently.

If your child has to take medications to school, he may be embarrassed about using them in front of other kids. Children can be cruel and may tease your child.

If possible, have your child's doctor adjust the medication schedule so that she takes most doses at home.

> If your child is faced with the prospect of taking medication at school, talk with your child's teacher, principal, and school nurse to make the delivery of the medication as inconspicuous as possible.
>
> —Marc S. McMorris, M.D.,
> Mott Children's Hospital
> at the University of Michigan

Teens

Once your child hits adolescence, refusing to take her medication may become part of the normal rebellion that goes on at this age. Don't give up. Try to make her understand that failing to keep her asthma under control could mean that she ends up in the hospital's ICU one night—or worse. Perhaps remind your child that even though taking the medication is inconvenient, having uncontrolled asthma is even more inconvenient.

> If your child has been neglecting his medication and has recently been sick because of it, calculate how much time he lost during the illness. He may have been in the hospital for a week and recovering for several more days at home. Compare this to the two or three minutes a day it takes to keep this from happening with preventive medications. Adding all this up can be quite persuasive.
>
> —STEVEN KANENGISER, M.D., F.A.A.P., F.C.C.P.,
> ST. JOSEPH'S MEDICAL CENTER,
> PATERSON, NEW JERSEY

These trips to the hospital can be more than just inconvenient. The drugs that are used when your child's asthma gets out of control are much more potent than his regular medications.

> Remind your child that if they neglect their preventive medicines, they will end up having acute asthma attacks and will have to use medications that can make them feel jittery or hyper. This will sometimes get them back on track.
>
> —MARC S. MCMORRIS, M.D.,
> MOTT CHILDREN'S HOSPITAL
> AT THE UNIVERSITY OF MICHIGAN

Steroids

The use of steroids in asthma medications worries parents almost as much as their child's asthma. The word "steroids" is associated in many people's minds with nasty side effects, and we've all heard about athletes who harm their bodies and athletic careers trying to pump themselves up.

However, while inhaled steroids do have some side effects, they are much different from the form athletes illegally inject into their muscles. The dosages are much smaller, and the medication is delivered directly into the lungs. While the side effects are still being studied, and researchers have reported some slowing of growth in patients using steroids, children generally reach normal height by adulthood.

Still, these medications are not to be taken lightly, and the quest for an effective asthma medication with no side effects is ongoing.

To help minimize the side effects from asthma medications with steroids:

- Work with your child's doctor to find the minimum dose of steroids that is effective in controlling your child's asthma.
- Make sure your child uses a spacer when taking a steroid inhaler. This helps limit the amount of medication deposited in the mouth.
- Make sure your child rinses her mouth immediately after using a steroid inhaler. One way to ensure this is to have her use the inhaler right before brushing her teeth, morning and night.

—STEVEN KANENGISER, M.D., F.A.A.P.,
F.C.C.P., ST. JOSEPH'S MEDICAL CENTER,
PATERSON, NEW JERSEY

Doctors report that children with poorly controlled asthma don't grow well, and that uncontrolled asthma can lead to irreversible "remodeling" of the airways and permanent lung damage. Steroids are among the very best anti-inflammatory medications available to prevent both of these occurrences. Using these preventive medications as directed can lessen the impact of your child's asthma and help her lead a more normal life.

ADJUST YOUR ATTITUDE

Your attitude toward your child's asthma can be a major factor in how he or she perceives the disease. Doctors report that parents often have trouble accepting that their child has asthma and treat the diagnosis as a tragedy. There's no reason a child with asthma should not lead a normal life.

> Think of it this way: You don't have an asthmatic child, you have a child with asthma. They're children first.
> —MARY ANN LEWIS,
> MATTEL CHILDREN'S HOSPITAL AT UCLA

Too much negativity about the disease and your child won't feel comfortable telling you about her symptoms or any attacks she may have had. This means that information won't get to her doctor, and he won't be able to properly help manage the disease. Your child will also be more likely to resist treatment. In other words, your negative attitude could make your child's asthma worse. The more relaxed and matter-of-fact you are about your child's condition, the more she is apt to perceive it as "no big deal." This will help her see that if her asthma is under control, she can get on with the business of being a kid.

To help your child have a good attitude toward treatment, good treatment goals are essential. Many doctors express treatment goals—measurements of how much they hope to improve your child's condition—in terms of readings on a peak-flow meter or some other clinical measure of lung function. This tracks progress quite accurately for the doctor, but it's meaningless to your child.

> Ask your child to name three things he can't do because of his asthma, or things his condition causes that he doesn't like. Then you can work with your doctor to turn these things into treatment goals. Examples of goals might include being able to play basketball without having an attack, missing fewer days of school, or taking fewer trips to the hospital.
>
> —RICK VINUYA, M.D.,
> CHILDREN'S HOSPITAL OF MICHIGAN

This kind of goal is not only more meaningful to your child, it will help give him a real sense of participation in the treatment and a sense of control over his asthma.

WHEN TO CALL THE DOCTOR

Each child with asthma has specific conditions that merit a call to the doctor. Your individual asthma action plan, which you'll need to work out in advance with the doctor, should clearly explain what these conditions are for your child.

However, if you're in doubt, doctors generally prefer that you call sooner rather than later. Calling with a question about which medication to use, or confirming dosage instructions, is better than leaving things unclear and having to meet the doctor later in the emergency room.

Keep in mind that asthma can be unpredictable. No matter how well you and your child work to manage the disease, things can happen that will catch you off guard. In these cases, follow your instinct to call your doctor or visit the hospital immediately—even if the specifics of this situation aren't covered in your action plan.

Athlete's Foot

It isn't a serious problem, but it can be . . . uncomfortable. Athlete's foot is caused when a fungus infects the skin of the foot and grows in the warm, moist environment inside shoes and socks. There are three basic forms of the condition. The first and most common appears on the webbing between the toes. The second is the "moccasin" type, which affects the bottom and sides of the foot. The third, known as the bullous type, consists of moist blisters in the webs of the toes and on the soles and instep of the foot.

Athlete's foot, technically called tinea pedis, is uncommon in preadolescent children and more likely to be found in preteen or teenage kids who are athletic or spend lots of time wearing sneakers. If you have a young child with foot problems, see your doctor.

Don't use over-the-counter athlete's foot preparations on kids under age ten before seeing your doctor. These treatments may make the child's true condition more difficult to diagnose.

—LORETTA DAVIS, M.D.,
MEDICAL COLLEGE OF GEORGIA

In a younger child, what looks like athlete's foot could be foot eczema, which causes excessive drying of the skin; psoriasis; or even contact dermatitis from an allergic reaction to the materials in the child's shoes or socks. Treatments for athlete's foot will be basically ineffective in these cases; a visit to the doctor will provide an accurate diagnosis and quicker treatment.

FIRST RESPONSE

OVER-THE-COUNTER MEDICATION

Doctors report that over-the-counter athlete's foot medications tend to be effective with older kids and adults, and are worth trying even before you see the doctor. Just make sure you choose a medication made specifically for fungal infections of the foot. The most common types contain miconazole (Micatin), clotrimazole (Lotrimin or Mycelex), and tolnaftate (Aftate for Athlete's Foot, Tinactin) as their active ingredients, and come as powders and creams.

Creams work best for treating ongoing athlete's foot infections and should be applied as a thin layer to help keep the foot as dry as possible. Powders tend to be better for preventing recurrent cases and can be used for a longer period of time because they also help keep the foot dry.

—SHEILA FALLON FRIEDLANDER, M.D.,
CHILDREN'S HOSPITAL SAN DIEGO

These preparations are fungistatic, which means they keep the fungus from reproducing but don't kill it; the infection will be over when the existing fungus dies out.

> For over-the-counter medications to be effective against athlete's foot, you must continue treatment for a week or two after the last of the fungus is totally gone, to make sure you have neutralized any remaining trace. Most people stop treatment too early and the condition comes back.
>
> —LORETTA DAVIS, M.D.,
> MEDICAL COLLEGE OF GEORGIA

Over-the-counter products should clear up a case of athlete's foot in one to three weeks. The moccasin-type athlete's foot may respond less quickly because it involves a larger area and so a greater amount of fungus. If the infection is still around after three weeks, see your doctor.

> Stop using over-the-counter athlete's foot products immediately if your child's condition seems to worsen. Your child could be allergic to something in the medication.
>
> —JANICE YUSK, M.D.,
> KOSAIR CHILDREN'S HOSPITAL,
> LOUISVILLE, KENTUCKY

One thing you should *not* use on any form of athlete's foot is cortisone cream. Cortisone may stop the itch temporarily, but it actually encourages the fungus to grow and could make the condition worse.

COMFORT CARE

While a mild case of athlete's foot may not cause your child much discomfort at all, more severe cases can cause plenty of itch and even pain if the skin begins to crack. Many of the measures that make a case of athlete's foot more comfortable will also help heal the condition and keep it from coming back.

ITCH, ITCH, ITCH

The most talked-about symptom of athlete's foot is the itch. Over-the-counter medications can take weeks to work, but doctors report that the itch usually subsides after a few days. In the meantime, here are a few tricks to help get your child's mind off her feet.

> If the itching is uncomfortable, choose a powdered athlete's foot medication rather than a cream. These help absorb moisture, keeping the foot dry and reducing the itch.
>
> —LORETTA DAVIS, M.D.,
> MEDICAL COLLEGE OF GEORGIA

> Try soaking the feet in cool water or a combination of Burrows solution and cool water. The salt content of the Burrows solution will help dry out the fungus.
>
> —PETER COLE, M.D.,
> PHOENIX CHILDREN'S HOSPITAL

Cool compresses can also be used for ten to fifteen minutes at a time, three to four times a day. Doctors report that Burrows solution (aluminum acetate) tends to be especially effective against wet, blistering infections.

For cases of extreme itching that is keeping your child awake, give a dose of oral antihistamine like Benadryl. This will ease the itching and help make your child drowsy.

—Sheila Fallon Friedlander, M.D.,
Children's Hospital San Diego

CLEAN AND DRY

One important part of clearing up a case of athlete's foot is to keep the feet clean, especially the area between the toes. Wash away as much of the fungus as possible, and don't give it any place to take hold.

Wash the foot gently with antibacterial soap, and use an antibacterial cream like Polysporin on any open sores to help prevent secondary bacterial infection.

—Janice Yusk, M.D.,
Kosair Children's Hospital,
Louisville, Kentucky

To help clean the foot and fight the bacteria, wash with a soap containing benzoyl peroxide, the same active antibacterial ingredient found in many acne treatments. It might also help to use an over-the-counter acne treatment with benzoyl peroxide on the feet.

—Elliot F. Gellman, M.D.,
St. Louis Children's Hospital

But cleaning the foot will do no good if it stays moist enough for the fungus to continue spreading. Drying the foot and keeping it aired out is crucial.

If your child has an athlete's foot infection, have him dry his feet last after bathing or showering to prevent him from spreading the infection to other parts of the body.

—ELLIOT F. GELLMAN, M.D.,
ST. LOUIS CHILDREN'S HOSPITAL

Have your child use a blow dryer to dry her feet after bathing or showering—especially between the toes. This will ensure a thorough job.

—LORETTA DAVIS, M.D.,
MEDICAL COLLEGE OF GEORGIA

AIR IT OUT

One major cause of athlete's foot—especially among teens and preteens—are sneakers. Doctors call these "occlusive" footwear, which means they don't let the foot breathe. Some doctors report young patients who keep their prized tennis shoes on up to twenty hours a day.

As much as possible, have your child wear shoes that breathe, such as sandals or other open-toed shoes.

—DAVID LEFFELL, M.D.,
YALE–NEW HAVEN CHILDREN'S HOSPITAL

Choose light-colored sneakers and socks for your child with athlete's foot. Black ones tend to absorb the heat and hold it in.

—PETER COLE, M.D.,
PHOENIX CHILDREN'S HOSPITAL

Continue these measures as the infection clears. Remember that getting rid of the warm, moist environment around the foot means the fungus can't grow.

To help keep the feet cool and dry, use an antiperspi-
rant made especially for the feet, such as Drisol.

—Elliot F. Gellman, M.D.,
St. Louis Children's Hospital

FIGHT THAT FUNGUS

Once your child has weathered a case of athlete's foot, there's
a good chance she'll get it again. It even tends to run in families. Some doctors think it's because certain people are geneti-
cally predisposed, and others think it is simply that the fungus
spreads so easily. In any case, use preventive measures both
during and after a case of athlete's foot.

One way to prevent reinfection is to protect your child's
feet from exposure to the fungus as much as possible.

Have your child wear thongs, flip-flops, or rubber shoes
in public showers, locker rooms, and pools to keep
them from being exposed to fungus left on the floor by
other people with athlete's foot.

—David Leffell, M.D.,
Yale–New Haven Children's Hospital

You may also need to guard your child against exposure to
athlete's foot in other members of the family, and vice versa.

Spray a bleach-and-water solution or a bathroom
cleaner that contains bleach into the bottom of the
shower after any person in the family with athlete's foot
has used it. The bleach will kill any fungus left on the
surface.

—Janice Yusk, M.D.,
Kosair Children's Hospital,
Louisville, Kentucky

Using the powder or spray form of an over-the-counter athlete's foot treatment will fight the fungus and absorb moisture on the foot.

WHEN TO CALL THE DOCTOR

If over-the-counter treatment hasn't improved the condition at all after a few days, take your child to the doctor. Either the over-the-counter medication isn't up to the task, or your child has something else that requires a different type of treatment.

Go earlier if your child is experiencing severe discomfort or itch, or has breaks in the skin. This is especially true if your child has the type of athlete's foot that blisters. The doctor will likely be able to prescribe something to clear the infection more quickly than over-the-counter medications.

If your child has fever, swelling, redness, pus, or pain in the affected area, see your doctor immediately. This could mean that there is a secondary bacterial infection, which will need to be treated with antibiotics.

Blisters

A blister is really just a pillow. When the skin is injured by either friction or a burn, a pillow of liquid forms between its layers and protects the skin underneath while it heals. Children most often get blisters because of their growing feet. New shoes hardly seem broken in before they're already too small, and these too-small shoes rub against the foot and create friction blisters. The best thing you can do to prevent blisters is to keep an eye on your child's shoe size. Get your child's feet professionally measured and fitted at a shoe store rather than relying on the sizing gizmos at discount stores.

FIRST RESPONSE

TO POP OR NOT TO POP

If your child has a blister that is still intact, the first thing you're likely to wonder is whether you should pop it or leave well enough alone. This will depend on the size and location of the blister. The general consensus is that if the blister is small and painless, you should leave it intact.

Blisters caused by a burn—from a flame, hot surface, sunburn, or chemical—should never be popped. These get special treatment. See Burns.

> If a blister has been caused by a burn, hold it under cool water and then cover it with an over-the-counter burn ointment or cream.
>
> —JILL REEL, M.D., AND PATRICK STEINAUER, M.D.,
> BOYS TOWN NATIONAL RESEARCH HOSPITAL,
> OMAHA, NEBRASKA

However, you might want to consider popping the blister if:

- It's painful
- It's bigger than a dime
- It's in an area where there is likely to be continued friction, so that it would pop on its own anyway
- Your child has to continue walking, running, or participating in "the big game"
- The blister appears to be infected, with a red ring or red lines around it

COMFORT CARE

If you've decided to pop a blister, do it correctly. Otherwise you could do more damage or even cause an infection. If you're going to leave the blister intact, protect it properly so that it will stay intact. If it pops on its own, clean and bandage it so it can heal properly.

TO POP

When popping a blister, the first step is to clean the blister and surrounding skin with either antiseptic soap and water or rubbing alcohol. Then sterilize the needle. You can hold it under a flame, let it cool, and then wipe the black carbon residue away with a tissue, or use alcohol or bleach. Just be sure not to get the bleach on the skin.

> If you're sterilizing the needle by holding it under a flame, the part of the needle you are holding can become hot very quickly, so be careful.
>
> —STEPHEN WRIGHT, M.D.,
> KOSAIR CHILDREN'S HOSPITAL,
> LOUISVILLE, KENTUCKY

Once the needle and the skin are clean, gently puncture the blister.

> Pop the blister from the side, right at the edge, making a back-and-forth motion and a slit rather than a hole. If you just make one small hole, it can close up too easily, and then you have to puncture the blister again.
>
> —MARK DIDEA, M.D.,
> ARNOLD PALMER HOSPITAL FOR CHILDREN
> AND WOMEN, ORLANDO, FLORIDA

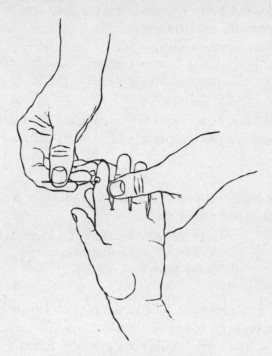

How to correctly pop a blister.

After you've punctured the blister, gently squeeze out the fluid. The blister is ready to bandage.

BROKEN BLISTERS

Gimme Some Skin

After you've popped a blister, or if it has burst on its own but the covering skin hasn't torn significantly, leave that skin intact. In these cases, just clean the blister thoroughly with soap (preferably antibacterial) and warm water, and cover it with a bandage.

Keep intact blisters covered until the dead skin on top begins to dry and flake away.

—Stephen Wright, M.D.,
Kosair Children's Hospital,
Louisville, Kentucky

If the burst blister has a flap of dangling dead skin loose, some doctors say to remove it, while others advocate leaving it alone.

If the blister pops open, cut off the dead skin to prevent infection and help it heal.

—Jill Reel, M.D., and Patrick Steinauer, M.D.,
Boys Town National Research Hospital,
Omaha, Nebraska

Dirt and germs can hide in the pockets left by the dead skin, and these are tough to clean out, especially in children. Taking off the extra skin is the surest way to get the blister clean, but this is a delicate operation your child may resist, and some doctors say that if you scrub the area thoroughly with soap and water, and bandage the blister with antibiotic ointment, the torn skin can be left alone.

The only time this skin should be left intact is if you are certain your child can keep the area completely clean.

—Caroline Chantry, M.D.,
University of California,
Davis Children's Hospital

If you do decide to remove the skin, explain to your child that you'll be cutting only dead skin that can't feel, so it won't hurt.

Carefully sterilize the scissors you use to cut away the skin, so that you don't cause infection.

—PHILIP OBIEDZINSKI, D.P.M., F.A.C.F.A.S.,
HACKENSACK UNIVERSITY MEDICAL CENTER,
NEW JERSEY

Make sure the scissors are sharp enough to cut the skin easily without tearing, and take care not to touch the patch of raw new skin underneath. This will hurt and might make your child flinch enough that you cut him.

Lift the dead skin gently with sterilized tweezers to make it easier to grasp. Cut it to the edge with the scissors, being careful not to cut into the undamaged skin.

—STEPHEN WRIGHT, M.D.,
KOSAIR CHILDREN'S HOSPITAL,
LOUISVILLE, KENTUCKY

Bandages

If a blister is broken or popped, the natural "bandage" it provides is gone. The vulnerable skin needs to be covered with antibiotic ointment, and bandaged for protection as it heals. Doctors advise against using hydrogen peroxide to clean wounds; it neither cleans away the dirt nor kills germs. The bandage should be kept clean and dry.

Change the bandage at least once a day and use antibiotic ointment, which will keep the bandage from sticking and damaging the area further. If the blister is oozing, change it more often. When a blister is broken, the skin underneath is left with no protection from infection.

—WILLIAM SHARRAR, M.D.,
CHILDREN'S REGIONAL HOSPITAL AT COOPER,
CAMDEN, NEW JERSEY

Doctors recommend avoiding ointments containing neomycin (an antibiotic): These are absorbed through the skin and can cause allergic reactions in some children.

Broken blisters should stay clean and covered until the new skin (the exposed part in the center of the blister) begins to dry and heal.

TO PROTECT

If you've decided not to pop an intact blister, your mission is to protect it from being popped before it is ready. The best way to do this is with good bandaging.

> Moleskin, corn pads, and Dr. Scholl's pads are all good forms of blister protection. Just leave space in the center for the blister, to take off the pressure.
> —PHILIP OBIEDZINSKI, D.P.M., F.A.C.F.A.S.,
> HACKENSACK UNIVERSITY MEDICAL CENTER,
> NEW JERSEY

Protect the blister until it pops on its own and the covering skin becomes dry and flakes away. This means the new skin underneath is healed and ready for exposure.

FOR THE PAIN

Until the new skin is completely healed, blisters are likely to be painful. Bandaging is certainly the best way to make sure the new skin is undisturbed, but there are other measures that will take away the hurt.

> Apply a cold compress as soon as possible after the blister is noticed.
> —RICHARD KENNEY, M.D.,
> SCOTTISH RITE CHILDREN'S MEDICAL CENTER,
> ATLANTA, GEORGIA

Doctors suggest you use cold compresses, rather than ice, which could damage the healing skin. A clean washcloth dipped in cold water is best, and should be held on for no more than twenty to thirty minutes. Some topical medications, such as Solarcaine, will also help.

Try giving an over-the-counter pain reliever like Tylenol to help with the pain.

—CAROLINE CHANTRY, M.D.,
UNIVERSITY OF CALIFORNIA
DAVIS CHILDREN'S HOSPITAL

STEPS TOWARD PREVENTION

The best way to avoid the pain of a blister is to avoid the blister itself. Aside from outgrown shoes, the most common cause of blisters are other types of friction (from sports, for instance, or if you are lucky enough to have an older child who does yard work) or burns.

If your child is going to be doing yard work, or some other activity involving friction on the hands, surgical-type gloves can help protect them. You can also tape areas you know are likely to blister.

—RICHARD KENNEY, M.D.,
SCOTTISH RITE CHILDREN'S MEDICAL CENTER,
ATLANTA, GEORGIA

Avoid wet shoes and socks. Wet friction is worst for creating blisters. Also make sure your kids break in their shoes.

—MARK DIDEA, M.D.,
ARNOLD PALMER HOSPITAL FOR CHILDREN
AND WOMEN, ORLANDO, FLORIDA

Basic burn prevention is a must, including keeping matches and flammable materials out of reach and always supervising children in the kitchen.

WHEN TO CALL THE DOCTOR

If your child has a blister that seems to be more than you can handle (it's very large, there are several together, or it's located on a joint), it's a good idea to see the doctor and have it checked out. You'll also want to visit the pediatrician in cases of large blisters caused by burns or chemical spills. Heat or chemical burns bad enough to blister merit medical attention.

If a blister is especially painful, even after it is popped, or has a bright red circle or red lines around it, it may be infected and might require antibiotics to clear things up. Blisters that develop a honey-colored crust may be caused by impetigo (a bacterial infection). These are both reasons to see the doctor.

Broken Bones, Sprains, and Strains

Half of all children break a bone before they reach adult-hood. Bones most likely to be involved are the fingers, collarbone, forearm, ankle, and nose. Doctors agree that fractures are much more common for kids under age ten than sprains, which are injuries to the ligaments around a joint. The growth plate, a thick layer of soft cartilage at the end of children's bones, is the weak link in a child's joint and is easily fractured. So if the swelling from what appears to be a sprain lasts more than a day or so, it may actually be a hairline fracture through the growth plate. This is as serious in a child as a broken bone in an adult. A common place for this type of fracture are the bones on the outside of the ankle, but it can also occur in the wrist and thumb. After age ten, children, like adults, are more likely to overstretch or tear ligaments, causing a sprain.

FIRST RESPONSE

ASSESSING THE INJURY

The first thing you should do after an accident serious enough to cause a fracture is to check for injuries to the head, neck, or spine. If you suspect an injury in any of these areas, don't attempt to move your child. Call an ambulance.

If the head, neck, or spine are not involved, you can turn your attention to the injured area. Doctors agree, however, that it can be extremely difficult to tell the difference between a break and a sprain in children, even with an X ray, because the growth-plate area of the joint shows as a dark spot on the X ray and tends to hide fractures.

If you suspect your child has a fracture, check for the following:

- Gross deformity of the limb
- Tenderness as you feel along the bones
- Numbness or tingling
- Abnormal color, temperature, or pulse in the affected area

If all else is normal, see if your child can move the affected limb. If it's a leg injury, see if she can put weight on it and take four steps. If all else is normal and the child has some use of the limb, it's probably not a fracture.

—Kurt Davey, M.D.,
Boys Town National Research Hospital,
Omaha, Nebraska

Seek immediate medical attention if there are any cuts near the injured area, since these could be the result of a bone fragment that poked through the skin. Injuries to the nose should be evaluated the same day by your pediatrician; she will check for septal hematoma, or bleeding inside the septum (the division between the nostrils). If bleeding is present and is not treated, the septum could become infected and cause irreparable damage to the nose.

If you suspect your child's injury is serious, call your pediatrician before giving any food or liquids of any kind; if the injury is severe enough to require surgery, your doctor will want your child's stomach to be empty prior to anesthesia. And even if you think your child's injury is minor, consult the pediatrician before giving pain reliever. Ibuprofen is recommended by doctors for sprains, since it helps reduce swelling, but acetaminophen is preferred for broken bones, since there is some evidence that ibuprofen can increase bleeding. Remember that in some cases, even doctors cannot be immediately sure whether or not a bone is broken. Don't give a child aspirin, which can lead to Reye's Syndrome in children, a rare but potentially serious complication.

COMFORT CARE

Sprains can generally be treated at home, without a trip to the doctor. Broken bones, on the other hand, require medical attention. In both cases your knowledge of first aid and the comfort care you provide during recovery can make even serious injuries much less painful and difficult for your child.

FIRST AID

Broken Limbs

If you suspect a broken bone your first step should be to immobilize the injury so that your child can be taken to the hospital. Doctors agree that splinting and immobilizing an injury will provide more pain relief than any medication. If any sharp fragments of a broken bone are allowed to move around, they could cut nerves or arteries, increasing the seriousness of the injury. If there is an obvious deformity, do not try to straighten out the bones: Just splint the limb as it is.

> One easy way to immobilize a break is to roll a magazine around the injured area and tape it in place. The magazine should be long enough to cover the entire injured area. Another way to immobilize an injury is to fluff a pillow, wrap it around the limb, and tape it in place.
>
> —ALVIN CRAWFORD, M.D.,
> CHILDREN'S HOSPITAL
> MEDICAL CENTER OF CINCINNATI

Immobilizing a broken bone with a rolled magazine.

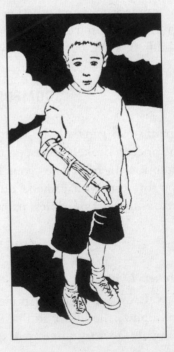

If you are making a splint using a rolled-up newspaper, wrap the limb with a pillow first to create a softer splint that allows room for additional swelling.

—DAVID SKAAGS, M.D.,
CHILDRENS HOSPITAL LOS ANGELES

If you don't have the material to make a splint, an injury to the arm can be immobilized by taping or strapping the arm to the chest. One mother I know immobilized her son's broken arm with a cookie sheet.

—ROBERT N. CLARK, M.D.,
CHILDREN'S HOSPITAL, COLUMBUS

If the injury involves the neck or head, or you think it will be impossible for you to splint the injury and keep the bones from moving, call an ambulance to take your child to the hospital. Don't move your child until the ambulance arrives. If the broken bones rub against each other, it will cause your child extreme pain. If you do take your child to the hospital by car, strap him into a car seat, booster seat, or seat belt as you normally would.

Broken Nose

Controlling your child's bleeding, which is common when the nose is injured, should be your first response.

To stop the bleeding, squeeze the soft part of your child's nose between your thumb and forefinger as your child leans forward. Hold this position until the bleeding stops. Having your child lean forward keeps him from breathing in blood that might run down the back of the throat.

—DONALD B. KEARNS, M.D., F.A.A.P., F.A.C.S.,
CHILDREN'S HOSPITAL SAN DIEGO

Once the bleeding has stopped, apply ice to help decrease the swelling. Call your child's pediatrician to make an appointment and find out whether you can give acetaminophen for pain. Doctors recommend against ibuprofen in such cases, as it is likely to increase bleeding.

If there is no septal hematoma (or bleeding in the septum), you will need to return to the doctor only if your child can't breathe through the nose or if it's become deformed. However, the swelling will take at least a week to decrease enough for the doctor to evaluate and treat these complications.

Cases of cosmetic deformity must be treated within three weeks of injury to the nose or it will heal improperly and may necessitate plastic surgery. In cases where the break is not severe, the nose is simply maneuvered back into proper position and splinted for about a week.

Sprains

If you suspect a sprain, get the swelling down to relieve pain, and rest the injured area so it can heal. You can remember the correct first aid using the acronym RICE (rest, ice, compression, elevation). Apply ice packs to the injured area, bandage the injury, and keep it elevated. Make sure your child doesn't use the affected limb, and if the injury hasn't improved in three days, call your doctor.

Apply ice packs for about twenty minutes every hour. Bags of frozen vegetables will do in a pinch. Use a protective barrier, such as a washcloth, between the ice and your child's skin. If your child tells you the pack is getting too cold, remove it and reapply later.

—KURT DAVEY, M.D.,
BOYS TOWN NATIONAL RESEARCH HOSPITAL,
OMAHA, NEBRASKA

Have two refreezable ice bags available, so one is ready for use while the other is being refrozen.

—ROBERT J. BIELSKI, M.D.,
LOYOLA UNIVERSITY MEDICAL CENTER

When wrapping a sprained arm or leg, make sure you can see your child's fingers or toes. This will help you make sure the bandages aren't too tight. A child with a properly wrapped injury should be able to move her fingers or toes. If she can't, or if there is any discoloration, numbness, or swelling of the fingers or toes, the injury is wrapped too tightly. The bandages should be removed immediately and reapplied.

—ALVIN CRAWFORD, M.D.,
CHILDREN'S HOSPITAL MEDICAL CENTER
OF CINCINNATI

The injured area must be above the heart for proper elevation of an injury. Though it may be difficult to keep your child in the right position, it's worth the effort, since this will decrease swelling and pain.

To keep your child's injured leg elevated at night, place couch cushions at the lower end of the bed between the mattress and box springs. This will elevate the entire bottom of the mattress and will keep your child from kicking the pillow out from underneath the leg during sleep.

—DAVID SKAAGS, M.D.,
CHILDRENS HOSPITAL LOS ANGELES

If your child's condition begins to improve within a day or two, there is probably no need to take her to the doctor.

RECOVERY

While your child is recovering, you should extend your first-aid measures—rest, ice, compression, elevation for sprains; rest and elevation for broken bones—for as long as they prove helpful.

Pain Medication

Resting and elevating the injury helps keep the swelling down and lessens the need for medication, but a child with a serious sprain or a broken bone almost always requires some. Doctors commonly prescribe Tylenol with codeine; headache is one common side effect of codeine. If your child gets such a headache, discontinue her pain medication immediately and give an over-the-counter headache remedy such as ibuprofen or acetaminophen. Then contact your pediatrician and ask her to prescribe an alternative pain reliever.

Other side effects of codeine include nausea, vomiting, drowsiness, light-headedness, and constipation. Ibuprofen will sometimes provide the same relief as narcotic medications without many of these side effects. It can, however, cause upset stomach.

> If your child has nausea with codeine or ibuprofen, offer simple foods such as clear liquids and crackers. Avoid heavy, greasy foods.
>
> —RICHARD M. SCHWEND, M.D.,
> CHILDREN'S HOSPITAL OF BUFFALO

Constipation from codeine can be treated using dietary fiber, fruits, and juices (see "Constipation"). Drowsiness is a lesser worry. Doctors agree that a child who is in enough pain to require codeine shouldn't be in school or leave the house for other activities. This allows plenty of time to stay home and rest.

Coping with a Cast

If your child experiences excessive pain or swelling while wearing a cast, consult your pediatrician. Also see the doctor if a cast begins to show signs of wear at joints like the heel or elbow, loosens, or breaks. Less serious problems can be dealt with at home.

Central Casting

No matter the type, casts come in two parts—the inner layer of padding that is rolled around the injured area, and the hard outer shell. While most cast padding is the same, there are several types of shells that might be used in your child's cast.

PLASTER OF PARIS

This is the traditional white cast. It is made of strips of plaster-impregnated bandaging that are soaked in water, applied to the injury, then allowed to dry.

Advantages
This cast is breathable, so it doesn't retain as much heat and moisture. It's also less expensive and easier to work with than other types of casts.

Disadvantages
Plaster of paris casts are heavier than other types of casts. They are also less durable and cannot get wet—even a little.

Care
This type of cast should be kept dry and as clean as possible. If it does get wet, try drying it with a blow dryer on a cool setting. If this doesn't work, call your doctor. If your child has a plaster leg cast, she shouldn't walk on it unless her doctor has specifically told her it is okay.

(continued)

FIBERGLASS

This type of cast is created with strips of fiberglass-impregnated bandaging, which are dipped in water, wrapped around the padding, and allowed to dry. These are sometimes used with a waterproof Gore-Tex liner.

Advantages
These lightweight, durable casts are water-resistant and ten times more durable than plaster casts. If they have a Gore-Tex liner, they are even okay for swimming. They are also available in a wide variety of bright colors and patterns.

Disadvantages
These casts do not breathe, so they tend to make the limb hot and sweaty. They are also more difficult to apply than plaster, so they may not be suitable for all types of injuries. Gore-Tex liners tend to wear out after three weeks and are not appropriate for casts that must stay on for longer periods of time. If a Gore-Tex–lined cast gets wet and isn't dried out properly, it can cause severe blistering of the skin.

Care
If your child's cast doesn't have a Gore-Tex liner, keep it dry. Casts with Gore-Tex liners must be dried with a blow dryer after getting wet.

SOFT CASTS

Called Scotchcast Softcast, these casts are made of knitted fiberglass impregnated with polyurethane, but the material is slightly less rigid than other types of fiberglass casts.

Advantages
These casts can be peeled off, so your child is spared the fright of the cast saw.

Disadvantages
Soft casts are not as rigid as other available types, so they may not be suitable for all injuries. Also, since they can be unwound, your child may decide to remove the cast himself.

Care
Keep the cast clean and dry, and prevent your child from unwinding or loosening it.

With all types of casts, doctors advise that you not let your child swim or bathe in a cast or walk on a leg cast unless the doctor has specifically said it's allowed. Sponge bathing is recommended. Showering in a cast is also okay if the limb can be double-wrapped in plastic and sealed above and below the cast with tape. You should also pay careful attention to any care instructions you received at the time the cast was applied.

Soreness

If you're elevating your child's broken leg, place the pillow under the calf, leaving the heel to hang free. The pressure from the pillow can create sores and blisters on the heel.

—ROBERT J. BIELSKI, M.D.,
LOYOLA UNIVERSITY MEDICAL CENTER

If your child experiences irritation or soreness at either end of the cast, moleskin, a type of padding used by hikers to fend off blisters, will often help. The material is self-adhesive and can be placed directly over any sore spots to protect them from further irritation. It's available at most drug- and sporting-goods stores.

—PAUL W. ESPOSITO, M.D.,
UNIVERSITY OF NEBRASKA MEDICAL CENTER

Itching: Itching is one of the most common problems associated with wearing a cast, and doctors agree that no matter how bothersome the itching, a child should never try to scratch by placing a pen, coat hanger, or other object under the cast. This can cause a nasty scratch or cut, and cuts underneath casts often become infected.

Oral Benadryl, which can be obtained without a prescription, can help with the itching. Your doctor may also be able to prescribe some medication for the itch.
—RICHARD M. SCHWEND, M.D.,
CHILDREN'S HOSPITAL OF BUFFALO

Avoid the beach and sandbox if your child is wearing a cast, and don't attempt to stop the itching with powders. Sand particles can get trapped under the cast and drive the patient crazy with itching. Powders, when mixed with sweat, turn into a thick goo, which can actually increase itching. Instead, try blowing cool air under the cast with a blow dryer on a cool setting, or sucking cold air through the cast with the thin corner attachment of a vacuum cleaner.
—ROBERT J. BIELSKI, M.D.,
LOYOLA UNIVERSITY MEDICAL CENTER

Believe it or not, scratching the outside of the cast sometimes helps children deal with itching. Scratching the opposite limb in the same spot can also make the itching stop.
—PAUL W. ESPOSITO, M.D.,
UNIVERSITY OF NEBRASKA MEDICAL CENTER

Can't Write: If your child has a cast on the hand he uses to write, homework could become more of a chore than usual. Since a cast won't allow him to close his hand all the way, he'll find it difficult to hold a pen or pencil.

One option is to have your child try writing with the opposite hand, but this can take some practice.

If your child has a cast on her arm and can't hold a pen, try buying a novelty pen with a fat body, or wrapping a regular pen with plenty of tape to make it easier to hold.

—ROBERT J. BIELSKI, M.D.,
LOYOLA UNIVERSITY MEDICAL CENTER

Choosing Crutches

Doctors prescribe crutches for both breaks and sprains when it's essential to keep weight off the affected limb in order for the injury to heal. However, children usually don't have the developmental skills to use crutches until they are at least five or six, about the time they develop the ability to ride a bike without training wheels. For smaller children, alternatives include walkers and wheelchairs.

If your child is old enough for crutches, choose child-size rather than adult-size models. Adjust them to your child's height, so the upper part of the crutch does not dig into his underarm. Your child's weight should rest on the heels of his hands, on the hand supports.

Watch to see that your child is using his crutches properly. If he's using the underarm rests to support his weight, he could end up with soreness or numbness under the arms. If his wrists aren't held straight, they may rub against the wooden supports and become sore.

—KURT DAVEY, M.D.,
BOYS TOWN NATIONAL RESEARCH HOSPITAL,
OMAHA, NEBRASKA

One of the biggest challenges to a child wearing crutches is learning to walk up and down stairs. A physical therapist may be able to provide some help here.

If your child has trouble learning to negotiate stairs on her crutches, she may be able to go up and down by sitting on each step and hoisting herself up or down with her arms. Let her.

—DAVID SKAAGS, M.D.,
    CHILDRENS HOSPITAL LOS ANGELES

Even though crutches can increase your child's mobility, plenty of rest and elevation are important to the healing process. Letting your child do too much too soon could delay recovery.

Having a Cast Removed

As frightening as breaking a bone can be for your child, removal of the cast can be even worse. The cast saw is loud, and children are understandably afraid it will cut *them* as well. Unfortunately, the cast saw is the only way to remove a plaster or fiberglass cast. Explaining a little about how the saw works will help calm your child's fears.

Refer to the device as a cast "remover," rather than a saw, to make it sound less frightening. Assure your child that the blade vibrates and does not spin. It will not cut off her limb. It may, however, burn the skin. To help prevent this, ask the person removing the cast to put a new blade on the saw.

—RICHARD M. SCHWEND, M.D.,
    CHILDREN'S HOSPITAL OF BUFFALO

Explain to your child that much of the noise that comes from the cast saw is really a vacuum cleaner that picks up the excess dust.

—ROBERT N. CLARK, M.D.,
    CHILDREN'S HOSPITAL, COLUMBUS

Using earplugs for your child can help lessen the noise of the cast saw and, with it, the fright.

—PAUL W. ESPOSITO, M.D.,
UNIVERSITY OF NEBRASKA MEDICAL CENTER

Headphones can mask the noise of the cast saw while providing a needed distraction during the removal of a cast.

—ROBERT J. BIELSKI, M.D.,
LOYOLA UNIVERSITY MEDICAL CENTER

Explain to your child that there is plenty of padding between the cast shell and his skin, and that this will help keep the saw from even touching his skin. Having your child talk with other children in the waiting room who have just had their casts removed may also help him be brave when facing cast removal.

—DAVID SKAAGS, M.D.,
CHILDRENS HOSPITAL LOS ANGELES

Doctors report that some children will be inconsolable despite their parents' best efforts and explanations. Most recommend that you stay with your child to offer comfort and support during the removal of the cast.

Regaining Motion

When a child is immobilized by a break or sprain, a temporary loss of some range of motion in the affected limb is common and generally not a cause for concern. Attempts to regain motion should be made only as your child is ready.

Adults, who take longer to heal than children and aren't generally as flexible, often need the help of a physical therapist. Children don't commonly require physical therapy unless the injury was severe enough to require surgery. However, parents are often asked to help their child do some exercises.

If the injury is a sprain, have your child gently trace the letters of the alphabet with the affected limb occasionally to help retain the full range of motion during recovery.

—DAVID SKAAGS, M.D.,
  CHILDRENS HOSPITAL LOS ANGELES

If your child has broken a limb, doctors recommend that you have your child start gently exercising the affected area as soon as the cast comes off and your pediatrician gives the okay. Once your child can resume normal activities, swimming is an excellent way to ease back into sports participation and strengthen the muscles.

To help your child regain full range of motion once a cast comes off, give hot baths to relax the muscles, then use gentle motion exercises. But go at your child's own pace. There is no need to restore full motion right away.

—DAVID SKAAGS, M.D.,
  CHILDRENS HOSPITAL LOS ANGELES

Before allowing your child to return to sports play, make sure she has normal motion and strength in the affected area. If the injury is to the leg, she should also be able to run forward and make a gentle "S" and a figure eight without pain or hesitation. She should also be able to run, cut and pivot, and perform all other motions she might perform during the sport.

—KURT DAVEY, M.D.,
  BOYS TOWN NATIONAL RESEARCH HOSPITAL,
  OMAHA, NEBRASKA

WHEN TO CALL THE DOCTOR

A child with a bad sprain or broken bone should be under a doctor's care. Contact your pediatrician immediately if your child's condition doesn't seem to be improving. Any of the following conditions also merit a call to the doctor:

- Your child's pain isn't relieved by elevation and medication
- The pain and swelling are not improving or have increased
- Your child experiences numbness, tingling, or weakness
- Your child has a high fever, pronounced redness around the limb, and excessive pain
- Your child has difficulty breathing

If there are no complications, just be sure to keep all follow-up appointments and follow your doctor's instructions. Eventually, the injured limb will return to normal. Children's bones heal quickly, and with a little time, your child should make a complete recovery.

Bruises and Black Eyes

When you're learning to make your way in the world, you're bound to encounter a few bumps. For kids, these are often accompanied by bruises or the occasional shiner. And while only time will bring back your child's true colors, there are a few things you can do to assure no greater damage has been done, and to make him more comfortable in the process.

FIRST RESPONSE

ASSESSING THE INJURY

Your first and most important indicator of the seriousness of the injury isn't how black-and-blue your child appears. It's the cause of the injury that likely will give you your best clue. If there's a bruise, you are looking for signs of a possible break or other serious injury. In cases of black eye, concussion and eye injury are your main concerns. Doctors recommend that you find out what caused the injury if you weren't there to see for yourself. Also be on the lookout for the following:

Concussion

Many black eyes are due to head injuries, rather than injuries to the eye itself. A blow to the upper part of the head or face may break blood vessels beneath the skin, and gravity will cause the resulting bruise to "leak" down and pool under the skin beneath the eye. If your child's injury was to the head, you must try to determine if she has suffered a concussion. Did your child lose consciousness or vomit at the time of the injury, or at any time since? Does she have a headache, or is she acting confused or unusually lethargic? Check to see whether her pupils are round and equal in size.

> When checking your child's pupils, shine a flashlight into the eyes. The pupils should both contract, and you only need to worry if there is a big difference in their size.
>
> —RICHARD KENNEY, M.D.,
> SCOTTISH RITE CHILDREN'S MEDICAL CENTER,
> ATLANTA, GEORGIA

You should also make sure your child isn't seeing double. If your child is too young to understand this concept, try holding up a toy and asking if she sees one, or more than one.

If you think your child might have suffered a concussion, call your doctor, who will probably give you instructions to observe your child carefully over the next twenty-four hours. This doesn't mean that you and your child can't get some sleep.

If you can't get your child to wake up and talk to you, or if she complains of severe headache, nausea, or vision problems, call the doctor.

You don't need to keep them awake, but check them about three hours after they go to sleep. Wake them and get them up for a glass of water so you can observe them. Ask about headache and double or blurred vision, and see if they can hold a normal conversation. If they're fine, there's no need to worry for the rest of the night.

—SAM SOLIS, M.D.,
CHILDREN'S HOSPITAL, NEW ORLEANS

Eye Injury

Another possibility if your child has a black eye is that the eye itself has been injured. Some of these injuries have fairly obvious signs, such as a foreign object in the eye, redness on the white of the eye or over the colored part of the eye (blood over the colored part of the eye is the greater cause for concern), or an eye that is swollen shut. Call your doctor or go to the emergency room in either case.

Other signs are more subtle. Can your child move her eyes up, down, right, and left? Have your child hold her head still and follow your finger with her eyes. Also find out if there is pain in the eye itself.

To help determine this in very young kids, who may not be able to tell you if the pain is *in* or *around* the eye, gently feel around the eye socket and ask them if that is the part that is hurting.

—ROBERT (BO) KENNEDY, M.D.,
ST. LOUIS CHILDREN'S HOSPITAL

You'll also need to figure out if your child can see normally out of both eyes. But simply asking your child if he can see okay isn't going to give you the answer. The uninjured eye will compensate for lack of vision in the other eye, so cover and check the vision in each eye to be certain.

> Your child should be able to see objects eighteen to twenty-four inches away. For a young child, you can hold up a small toy at the proper distance and see if she can identify it.
> —RICHARD KENNEY, M.D.,
> SCOTTISH RITE CHILDREN'S MEDICAL CENTER,
> ATLANTA, GEORGIA

You might think things would be easier with an older and more verbal child. But an older child is more likely to want to mask signs of poor vision to avoid a trip to the doctor or hospital. This means you'll need to take extra measures to make sure his vision is really all right.

> In an older child, don't just ask them whether they can see. Have them read something from the proper distance to get a more accurate measure of their vision.
> —CLEVE HOWARD, M.D.,
> MIAMI CHILDREN'S HOSPITAL

All cases of eye injury, however minor, are worth checking out with your doctor. If your child's vision is affected, you may also want to call your optometrist or ophthalmologist.

General Injury

If your child has a simple bruise on another part of the body, rather than a black eye, just make sure she hasn't broken, cut, or sprained anything in the bruised area. If a cut is involved, you have a whole different type of injury (see "Cuts"). Likewise, if your child isn't able to move or use the bruised body part without extreme pain, or if there is excessive swelling, there could be a break or sprain (see "Broken Bones, Sprains, and Strains").

If there is no concussion and/or the bruised body part still functions normally, you can go on and treat the bruise.

COMFORT CARE

RICE IS NICE

RICE—rest, ice, compression, and elevation—works well for treating many childhood injuries, but doctors say it is especially good for bruises. The "rest" part is usually simplest to achieve, as it isn't often that a child who has been seriously whomped in the eye or some other body part wants to continue running around. So encourage your child to take a breather, and to take it easy on the part or parts in question over the next few days.

Getting him to sit still for ice may be another matter, but icing should be done immediately to be effective. If you're out, don't wait until you get home. Get ahold of something cold and apply it to the bruised area.

> Ice isn't absolutely necessary. A washcloth soaked in ice-cold water is cold enough to do the job.
>
> —Heide Woo, M.D.,
> Mattel Children's Hospital at UCLA

According to physicians, one of the biggest mistakes parents make in treating a bruise is not slapping the cold stuff on right away. You don't need to make the area ice-cold, you just need to cool it down. Doctors say that a cold steak or other piece of beef isn't any more effective than other, cheaper options. In fact, other food groups make good alternatives.

A bag of frozen peas or corn is most practical. It is readily available and easily conforms to the shape of the face.

—ROBERT (BO) KENNEDY, M.D.,
ST. LOUIS CHILDREN'S HOSPITAL

Most doctors, however, are happy with the classic bag of ice.

Ice should be applied within twenty to thirty minutes of the injury. Try adding water to your plastic bag of ice, so that it will better conform to the contours of the face or body.

—DOLORES MENDELOW, M.D.,
MOTT CHILDREN'S HOSPITAL
AT THE UNIVERSITY OF MICHIGAN

No matter what you use, if it's frozen, experts warn not to put it directly on the skin—especially around the eye. All bags of ice or other things from the freezer should first be insulated with a cloth. The cold stuff basically helps contract the broken blood vessels that are feeding into the bruise and so helps minimize the discoloration. It can also help with swelling and pain for the same reasons.

Wetting the cloth you use to cover your ice pack helps distribute the cold quickly and evenly.

—SAM SOLIS, M.D.,
CHILDREN'S HOSPITAL, NEW ORLEANS

Rig a bandana to hold the ice in position so your child can play. If she has a black eye, you can turn her into a pirate.

—RICHARD KENNEY, M.D.,
SCOTTISH RITE CHILDREN'S MEDICAL CENTER,
ATLANTA, GEORGIA

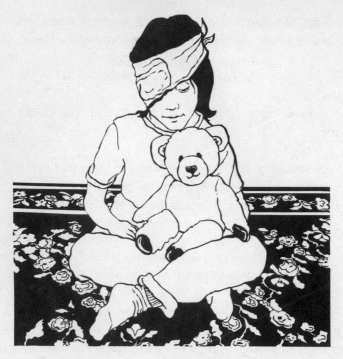

Using a bandana "pirate style" to hold an
ice pack over a black eye.

If your child resists the ice despite your efforts, it probably isn't worth the trouble, and could even make the child
feel worse.

If a child is upset about having ice put on him or her and
putting more cloth between the ice and the child doesn't
help, the best thing to do is to put the ice back in the ice-
box. A screaming child is not a resting, calm child.

—NATHAN HAGSTROM, M.D.,
CONNECTICUT CHILDREN'S MEDICAL CENTER

Use ice packs or cold compresses for the first twenty-four hours after the injury to help reduce bruising, swelling, and pain. The ice also helps to distract an upset child immediately after the injury. You might also try massaging an area away from the bruise.

> A gentle kiss to the bruise has an excellent placebo effect on children.
>
> —Nathan Hagstrom, M.D.,
> Connecticut Children's Medical Center

Using compression, or gentle pressure with the ice pack, also helps stop or slow the leakage of blood from the broken vessels into the bruise. Doctors recommend icing and compression three to four times a day, for ten to twenty minutes each time, or whatever your child will tolerate.

The final part of the RICE plan is elevation. Keeping the injured area elevated above the heart helps minimize swelling and pain, especially in the area around the eye. If your child has a black eye or a bad bruise, try having him sleep with the injured area elevated. In a case of black eye, he doesn't need to be completely upright; the head just needs to be above the heart, so an extra pillow should do the trick. Doctors say, however, that it isn't worth the trouble to elevate a minor bruise.

If your child has a black eye and you don't elevate his head, the swelling may be worse the following morning. Lying flat keeps the fluids from draining away. This additional swelling should go down around thirty minutes after he gets up.

OVER-THE-COUNTER

You can give your child an over-the-counter pain reliever if the ice doesn't seem to be enough. Most doctors prefer acetaminophen (the active ingredient in Tylenol). Some say ibuprofen (Motrin) is fine to use, though it won't minimize the bruising because it thins the blood. Most doctors warn against giving aspirin to children without consulting a pediatrician.

> Avoid sedating medications, especially in cases of head injury. They can make the seriousness of the injury tough to evaluate.
> —SAM SOLIS, M.D.,
> CHILDREN'S HOSPITAL, NEW ORLEANS

Most doctors maintain that over-the-counter eyedrops won't help in cases of black eye.

LOOKIN' AT YOU

If there is no underlying injury, bruises and black eyes generally tend to look much worse than they really are. Pain and swelling from a bruise shouldn't last long after the initial injury, and much of the remaining treatment is for cosmetic reasons. Once you've used RICE to minimize the bruising, swelling, and pain during the first twenty-four hours, some doctors recommend applying heat to help the bruising go away.

> Apply moist heat four times a day for twenty minutes to help clear away the blood that has pooled under the skin.
> —RICHARD KENNEY, M.D.,
> SCOTTISH RITE CHILDREN'S MEDICAL CENTER,
> ATLANTA, GEORGIA

Some doctors say that this won't help enough to be worth the trouble, and that you should bother only if it makes your child feel better. In any case, the bruise or black eye will likely progress through its purple stage to black-and-blue, brown, and yellow-green before it goes away in about two weeks.

If you have a preschooler or elementary-age child with a black eye, talk to her teacher about it before sending her back to class. Her appearance may frighten the other kids, or it may get her teased. The teacher can help prevent this.

—Dolores Mendelow, M.D.,
Mott Children's Hospital,
at the University of Michigan

WHEN TO CALL THE DOCTOR

BLACK EYES

- If your child shows signs of an injury to the eye itself
- If your child won't cooperate and let you examine her eye, or can't tell you how she was injured
- If the pain comes back after the initial injury: this could be a sign of bleeding into the eye, or swelling inside the eye
- If your child develops a fever: this could be a sign of infection from a previously unnoticed cut to the eyelid

BRUISES

- If there is another injury in addition to the bruise itself
- If the bruise is bigger than your hand or keeps growing: This could be a sign of a bleeding disorder
- If the bruise doesn't heal in about fourteen days: Again, this could be a sign of a bleeding disorder

Burns

Burns are one of the leading causes of accidental death in childhood, according to the Nemours Foundation, and are second only to motor vehicle accidents. To help keep your child safe, doctors recommend that you take basic childproofing measures, such as locking matches, lighters, flammable liquids, and other chemicals out of reach. You should also never let a child under age ten use a stove or other cooking appliance unsupervised. Because many serious burns are from hot water, doctors also recommend that you set your household water heater no higher than 120 degrees Fahrenheit, and keep pot handles on the stove turned in when cooking.

FIRST RESPONSE

COOL IT DOWN

Your first concern if your child has suffered a burn is to cool the burn quickly to help reduce damage to the skin and underlying tissue. The best way to do this is with cool running water.

> If you don't have running water available, put the burn in contact with another cool liquid if you can.
> —JOAN SHOOK, M.D.,
> TEXAS CHILDREN'S HOSPITAL

If your child suffers a chemical burn, flush the area with lots of running water. If the burned area is larger than your palm, phone for emergency medical help and continue to flush the burned area while you wait for help to arrive. If the area is small, bandage it loosely after ten to twenty minutes and call your child's doctor.

Never apply ice or ice packs to any kind of burn, as this could further damage the skin.

You can often tell by the appearance how serious a burn is.

- First-degree burns look like a sunburn. They are just mildly red.
- Second-degree burns have some blistering.
- Third-degree burns involve the full thickness of the skin. The skin may look pale or charred. These burns may not be painful, because the nerve endings in the skin are damaged. These always require medical attention.

If your child suffers an electrical burn, the skin may appear only slightly damaged at the surface, but may be burned more seriously underneath. Seek medical attention immediately. Electrical burns to the mouth can leave severe scarring.

> If the skin from a burn is blistered, the blistered skin doesn't likely feel pain. The pain sensation comes from the area around the blistered skin. Put cold compresses around, rather than on, the blisters.
>
> —FRANCISCO MEDINA, M.D.,
> MIAMI CHILDREN'S HOSPITAL

> Have a first-aid chart in your home so that it can ground you in times of stress, such as when your child is hurt. The chart will tell you exactly what you need to do, and you won't have to kick yourself later because you forgot something.
>
> —JOAN SHOOK, M.D.,
> TEXAS CHILDREN'S HOSPITAL

Once you have the burn cooled off, most minor burns— including almost all first-degree and smaller second-degree burns—can be treated at home.

COMFORT CARE

If you keep the skin clean and can treat any pain your child may have, your child won't need medical attention for a minor burn.

COMING CLEAN

It is important to get burned skin clean in order to prevent infection, but be careful not to use harsh soaps or detergents, which will irritate the skin. Use hand soap or the most mild soap you have in the house.

Do not put lemon juice, iodine, vinegar, or any other strong
substance on a burn. This will further irritate the skin.

—FRANCISCO MEDINA, M.D.,
MIAMI CHILDREN'S HOSPITAL

Don't put butter on the burn or apply other home remedies. They can be dirty and introduce infection. They can
also trap the heat.

Blisters provide some cushioning and protection for the
damaged skin underneath, so don't pop them. Instead, cover
them with a light gauze dressing to protect them. The blister
provides a sterile dressing for the burn. After the blisters have
popped, dress them with a bandage and Polysporin. (see
"Blisters")

BABY-BURNED SKIN

Minor burns without blisters don't need to be bandaged,
but sometimes bandaging helps with the pain, according to
doctors.

To bandage a burn, wrap three or four layers of gauze
around it loosely and tape it to the skin below and
above the burn.

—JOAN SHOOK, M.D.,
TEXAS CHILDREN'S HOSPITAL

Do not use cotton when bandaging a burn. The fibers will
stick to the skin and be very difficult to remove later.

—FRANCISCO MEDINA, M.D.,
MIAMI CHILDREN'S HOSPITAL

You can also apply a topical burn cream or pain reliever
such as Solarcaine, or give your child Motrin or Tylenol for
pain. If keeping the burn in cool water feels good, that's okay,

too, though doctors say cool water isn't likely to feel good after the first hour or so.

> Toothpaste, vitamin A cream, Vaseline, or any other mild, cool cream can help relieve the pain of a burn once the burned skin has been cooled down with water or cool compresses. The fewer chemicals the cream has in it, the better, as chemicals might irritate the burned skin.
>
> —FRANCISCO MEDINA, M.D.,
> MIAMI CHILDREN'S HOSPITAL

WHEN TO CALL THE DOCTOR

Third-degree burns always require medical attention. You should also call your child's doctor if your child has a burn on the hands, feet, or genital area, or has a burn that is bigger than your palm. You should also seek medical attention for an infant with a burn of any sort, or for a child with a second-degree burn to the face.

If you are treating a minor burn at home and your child still has severe pain an hour after the proper dose of Tylenol, your doctor might be able to prescribe something to relieve it. If a burn you are treating becomes redder, swollen, and tender, with a pus-like coating, it is likely infected, and your child will need antibiotic treatment. Seek medical attention.

Canker Sores
and Fever Blisters

They begin with a tiny tingle or a little blister—a sore barely visible on your child's lip or inside her mouth. Canker sores and fever blisters (also known as cold sores) have tormented us throughout history (an epidemic of fever blisters caused the emperor Tiberius to ban kissing in ancient Roman public ceremonies), and we still don't know how to cure them. They pain and embarrass adults, but they can keep children from eating, drinking, and sleeping . . . reducing both parent and child to the point of tears.

Canker sores and fever blisters are often confused. Though they both cause pain, and appear in and around the mouth, they are really two different types of sores with different causes and courses of healing.

Canker sores appear inside the mouth—usually on the tongue, the inside of the cheeks, the soft palate, and the base of the gums. No one knows what causes them. These crusty little sores are not contagious, and the pain generally decreases in seven to ten days, with complete healing in one to three weeks.

Fever blisters usually show up around the mouth, but they can also appear on the roof of the mouth or upper part of the gums. They are caused by the herpes virus (though not the same one that causes genital herpes) and are highly contagious. Many children who have them, in fact, were infected by their parents or other caregivers—people who usually give lots of kisses. Children, in turn, spread the virus to one another by touching the sores and then other children. Fever blisters appear first as small blisters, which then burst and turn into sores. They usually heal within two weeks.

FIRST RESPONSE

WHICH SORE IS IT?

If this is the first time your child has had mouth sores, and you have any doubts about what they are, see your doctor for diagnosis. In the meantime, treat them as contagious. If your child does have a fever blister, explain to her that she can spread it to other people, and she should try not to touch the sore or kiss others and should wash her hands often. You'll also need to resist the urge to kiss *her* anywhere near the mouth. Forehead kisses will have to do until the sore is completely healed.

COMFORT CARE

There is no reliable cure for either canker sores or fever blisters, and ways to shorten the course of healing are few. The best you can do is keep your child from irritating the sores further while they heal on their own, and make him as comfortable as possible. This is especially important; if the sores are severely painful, your child may not want to eat or drink enough, which could lead to dehydration.

PAIN MEDICATIONS

Some over-the-counter medications have proven fairly helpful against canker sores and fever blisters. Doctors report that acetaminophen, that good old standby, works well. You may also be tempted to try a local anesthetic like Orajel, but many doctors would prefer you didn't. Parents with a crying child on their hands may tend to overuse the medication, which can have serious side effects when not used as directed. The most dangerous of these include seizures, but the medications could also numb your child's gag reflex and cause choking. Even when used as directed, they can cause the child to bite the insides of his cheeks, which could bring on more sores.

Instead of Orajel, try using a half-and-half mixture of Benadryl (the pink, higher-strength oral suspension) and Maalox. Dab this on the sores with a cotton swab as needed. The Benadryl acts as an anesthetic to relieve the pain, and the Maalox helps coat the sores and protect them. It also reduces the acidity of the mouth. Because these are both designed to be taken orally, even if the mixture is dabbed on continually, your child won't get enough of either medication for an overdose.

—MICHAEL ZBIEGIEN, M.D.,
SUNRISE CHILDREN'S HOSPITAL,
LAS VEGAS, NEVADA

You can give Tylenol for the pain, or put something cold on the sores. Popsicles work well for canker sores, which are usually inside the mouth.

—HEIDE WOO, M.D.,
MATTEL CHILDREN'S HOSPITAL AT UCLA

Helpful ingredients of other over-the-counter preparations include glycerin, to protect the sore, and peroxide, to fight bacteria. Benadryl, whose main benefit is inducing sleep, can be used in severe cases but should be tried only with a doctor's recommendation. Another effective treatment against both types of sores is phenol (i.e. Campho-phenique), although ointments containing it are likely to burn when applied. Give your child a Popsicle prior to treatment, which may help numb the area, or will at least be a good bargaining tool for cooperation.

> Cold drinks, gelatin desserts, and Popsicles will all help numb the area and make kids more comfortable.
> —DONALD J. FILLIPPS, M.D.,
> SHANDS HOSPITAL, UNIVERSITY OF FLORIDA

> Saltwater rinses are worth a try to help promote healing. Mix half a teaspoon of salt with one cup of water. Be careful not to add too much salt or the solution may sting the sores. For older children, a solution of hydrogen peroxide and water is fine to use, but be careful, as your child shouldn't swallow peroxide.
> —DAVID BERGDAHL, M.D.,
> VALLEY CHILDREN'S HOSPITAL,
> MADERA, CALIFORNIA

AVOIDING IRRITATION

Both canker sores and fever blisters, no matter what might have caused them, are easily irritated. When sores are present, your child should avoid abrasive foods (pretzels, nuts, chips, hard candy), citrus, spicy, or hot foods. This probably won't be difficult to enforce. If your child refuses to listen, a single

sip of orange juice usually provides adequate "natural consequences" to get his attention.

Sun also tends to irritate mouth sores. Have your child
use a lip balm with sunscreen, which can prevent outbreaks
and might aid in healing by keeping existing sores from being
aggravated.

Also warn your child not to "mess with" either type
of sore. Canker sores, when irritated, only get worse and
can even leave scars. Fever blisters, because they are spread
through skin contact, can be transferred to others from your
child's hands, or can spread to their fingertips, creating something called a whitlow, an infection of the skin around the
fingernail that creates a painful open sore. The virus can also
cause an infection of the eye involving the eyelid and cornea.

To keep your child's mouth chemistry less acidic—as
saliva can be your child's own built-in irritant—make sure
she's taking in plenty of fluids. This can be difficult if mouth
pain is a problem, but it's essential. Cold beverages are best.

> If eating is painful for your child, try giving a Popsicle
> first. The cold will numb the sores and make eating
> easier.
>
> —Michael Zbiegien, M.D.,
>   Sunrise Children's Hospital,
>   Las Vegas, Nevada

GOOD ORAL HYGIENE

Keeping your child's mouth clean, and mouth sores clean and
dry, should ward off infection. Good oral hygiene is a must,
but toothbrushing can be painful with a mouthful of sores,
and overly enthusiastic brushing can even aggravate the problem (as can the minty-fresh flavor of many toothpastes).

If your child has trouble with the toothpaste, try dipping the toothbrush in plain baking soda for brushing instead.

—MICHAEL ZBIEGIEN, M.D.,
SUNRISE CHILDREN'S HOSPITAL,
LAS VEGAS, NEVADA

Another popular toothpaste ingredient, sodium laurel sulfate, can also aggravate or trigger sores, so look for a brand that doesn't contain it. And have your child go easy with that brush.

If your child is in too much pain for toothbrushing, it may not be worth the effort and could even cause further irritation. Instead, try a rinse with baking soda and water, which will help keep the mouth clean.

—DAVID BERGDAHL, M.D.,
VALLEY CHILDREN'S HOSPITAL

PREVENTION: DOWN IN THE MOUTH

The same things that irritate canker sores and fever blisters can also bring them on. If you've identified a trigger, ask your child to stay away from it even when there are no sores. Avoid injuring the inside of the mouth through hard foods and careless toothbrushing. Make sure your child's toothbrush has soft bristles, and remind her to chew foods slowly and carefully.

Have your child use a lip balm with sunscreen an SPF of at least 15 to help prevent outbreaks. Avoid extensive exposure to sunlight between ten A.M. and three P.M. when possible.

If your child has fever blisters and uses lip balm, make sure that particular tube or stick of lip balm is used only for that child, and only when he has an outbreak of sores. Have a different tube of lip balm to use when all the sores have healed. This will keep your child from spreading the sores, or from reinfecting himself.

—CANDACE JOHNSON, M.D.,
THE CHILDREN'S HOSPITAL, DENVER

Triggers—Shooting Your Mouth Off

If your child has recurring mouth sores, one way to avoid them is to determine what might have "triggered" the outbreak and help your child avoid it.

COMMON TRIGGERS FOR CANKER SORES

- Stress
- Skin injury (through hard foods like pretzels or potato chips, or careless toothbrushing by parent or child)
- Citrus, tomatoes, nuts
- Dietary deficiencies (iron, folic acid, or vitamin B12)
- Food allergies
- High-sugar foods

COMMON TRIGGERS FOR FEVER BLISTERS

- Emotional stress
- Illness, especially with fever
- Injury
- Exposure to sunlight
- Wind chapping
- Certain foods or food allergies

It is important to note that younger children are more likely to be triggered by illness, while older children may experience outbreaks at highly stressful times. When food is a trigger for either type of sore, the outbreak usually occurs within twenty-four hours of eating the offending food.

In the event of recurring sores, ask your child's doctor about blood and allergy tests to help determine whether a food allergy or dietary deficiency is contributing to outbreaks of cold sores.

WHEN TO CALL THE DOCTOR

If this is the first time your child has had mouth sores, see your doctor for a proper diagnosis and treatment.

For severe recurring cases of fever blisters, your doctor might prescribe Zovirax, which sometimes shortens the course of outbreaks if used within the first twenty-four hours after signs that an outbreak is coming. Zovirax is not widely used for children, as it requires that your child be able to recognize the earliest signs that a cold-sore outbreak is coming, according to David Bergdhal, M.D., of Valley Children's Hospital in California, and younger children can't alert parents in time for the medication to be effective. If you have cold sores yourself and have been prescribed acyclovir, don't give in to the temptation to use your prescription on your child.

Other reasons to call the doctor:

- If canker sores persist or recur more than two or three times per year
- If a mouth sore is larger than one centimeter, or lasts longer than two weeks (it may require medical treatment, including an antibiotic such as tetracycline)
- If your child has a mouth sore that has become infected
- If your child has mouth sores along with fever, diarrhea, headache, or skin rash
- If your child's entire mouth and gums are red

- If your child isn't drinking enough because of the mouth pain and becomes dehydrated

Pedialyte is good for fighting dehydration but tastes awful. To combat this, try mixing in one ounce of apple juice for every three ounces of Pedialyte to mask the taste. You can also add powdered, unflavored Pedialyte to other kinds of drink mixes your child likes.

—MICHAEL ZBIEGIEN, M.D.,
  SUNRISE CHILDREN'S HOSPITAL,
  LAS VEGAS, NEVADA

Chicken Pox

The biggest news about chicken pox is that soon there may not be any more. What was once considered a childhood rite of passage will likely be wiped out with the help of a vaccine that became available in 1995. The vaccine is recommended by doctors and the American Academy of Pediatrics, and is now an admission requirement in many public school districts. However, because it is new, there are still a fair number of cases of varicella (the other name for chicken pox) in children every year.

Since most cases aren't serious, children mainly need the care of a loving parent or other adult who knows a few tricks to help bring down fever and relieve itching.

The Chicken Pox Vaccine

In 1995, after more than ten years of research and clinical trials, the first chicken pox vaccine became available in the United States. Called Varivax, the vaccine has been shown to prevent illness in 70 to 90 percent of those who receive it. It is generally given in one injection to those twelve months or older, and it helps the body develop immune protection against the varicella-zoster virus.

Researchers haven't yet determined how long the vaccine continues to work. This is a concern for many people, as cases of adult chicken pox tend to be much worse than those contracted during childhood—especially if the adult in question is pregnant at the time of exposure. However, studies are ongoing to determine how long the immunity lasts, and experts expect to know soon whether a booster shot later in life will be required. Meanwhile, doctors continue to recommend that parents have their children vaccinated against chicken pox.

> The evidence so far is that the immunity lasts at least twenty years, and the benefits of the vaccine outweigh the risks of getting chicken pox as an adult. This is an illness worth preventing.
>
> JOSEPH DOCCHINI, M.D.,
> LOUISIANA STATE UNIVERSITY MEDICAL CENTER

Those who do get chicken pox after receiving the immunization generally have a milder illness with fewer lesions, according to studies. Varivax has generally been shown to be free of complications and was strongly recommended by every doctor I spoke with.

FIRST RESPONSE

NOT A TIME TO PARTY

There was a time when a mom who discovered her child had chicken pox invited all the other neighborhood children in to play so that they could be exposed and get their turn with the virus over with. At the very least, parents used to make sure siblings spent some time together so that they could weather the whole flock of chicken pox cases at once, rather than one at a time over a period of years.

The advent of the varicella vaccine has changed this approach substantially. Doctors now recommend that if one of your children comes down with chicken pox, you quarantine her as much as possible and get your other children vaccinated immediately (if they aren't already). Most cases of chicken pox are mild, but there are enough complications that doctors no longer consider it worth the risk to give children a case on purpose.

> Children who bring chicken pox into the household usually have a milder case, with fewer spots, than the siblings they give it to. If one of your kids gets chicken pox, it's a good idea to make sure the others are vaccinated.
>
> —MARK SCHLEISS, M.D.,
> CHILDREN'S HOSPITAL
> MEDICAL CENTER OF CINCINNATI

If you suspect your child has chicken pox, call the doctor and describe the symptoms. Your doctor will probably tell you *not* to bring your child into the office, says Ben Gitterman, M.D., of Children's National Medical Center. An uncomplicated case of chicken pox doesn't require medical attention, and the doctor won't want to risk spreading it to other patients.

If You Are Pregnant

If you are pregnant, have not had chicken pox, and are exposed to the virus, call your OB-GYN immediately. Approximately 90 percent of those who are not protected by an immunization and are exposed to the virus will come down with chicken pox, which could be serious during pregnancy. The illness can sometimes be prevented if the mother receives a dose of zoster immune globulin within twenty-four hours of exposure.

About 2 to 3 percent of pregnant women with chicken pox infect their infants in utero, which means the baby has chicken pox before it is even born, and the consequences can be severe. Pox in utero can cause extreme scarring or even the failure of a limb to develop if the virus is contracted during the first twenty weeks of gestation.

If the mother gets chicken pox toward the end of her pregnancy, she can infect her baby upon delivery. Chicken pox in newborns is serious and has a high mortality rate.

Due to the potentially serious consequences of chicken pox in pregnant women, and because the standard varicella vaccine cannot be given during pregnancy, doctors generally recommend that women of childbearing age who have not had chicken pox get the vaccination before becoming pregnant.

COMFORT CARE

An uncomplicated case of chicken pox generally makes a child itch; he will also have fever and general achiness.

DITCH THE ITCH

Skin Deep

Most treatments for mild itch—including calamine lotion and Aveeno oatmeal lotion—can be applied directly to the itching areas. As a basic, doctors recommend a tepid to cool bath at least once a day. This helps ease the itching and can also serve to keep the lesions (those endearing red spots) clean and prevent secondary infection.

> Use mild soap and water for your child's daily bath. Avoid products with artificial color or fragrance, and pat the skin dry afterward, rather than rubbing.
> —JOSEPH BOCCHINI, M.D.,
> LOUISIANA STATE UNIVERSITY MEDICAL CENTER

Adding oatmeal to your child's bath will also soothe the itch. You can add either regular oatmeal or one of the oatmeal bath products on the market. As with soap, just be sure the one you choose is free of artificial colors and fragrance.

Aside from cleaning and soothing, the bath also serves as a "dressing change" for an old chicken pox standby—calamine lotion. You probably remember your parents using it, and almost all doctors still recommend it to relieve the itch of chicken pox lesions. The calamine should be dabbed on gently with a cotton ball right after the bath; wash it off and reapply it after bathing each day. Otherwise, it could hold dirt and germs against the lesions. There are now clear brands of calamine in addition to the familiar peachy-pink.

> Don't use the type of calamine lotion that includes Benadryl. This allows the Benadryl to be absorbed through your child's skin and could lead to an overdose—especially if you are also giving Benadryl by mouth.
> —DEAN BLUMBERG, M.D.,
> UC DAVIS CHILDREN'S HOSPITAL

Scratching the lesions can lead to scars, and also to secondary infections if your child scratches hard enough to break the skin. Unfortunately, just telling your child not to scratch is rarely enough to stop her.

Put mittens or socks on your child's hands to keep them from scratching. You can make a game of this by turning the socks into sock puppets.

—MARK SCHLEISS, M.D.,
CHILDREN'S HOSPITAL
MEDICAL CENTER OF CINCINNATI

If the socks or mittens get pulled off, or if your older child balks at such measures, keep his nails trimmed and clean to reduce damage and the chance of secondary skin infection. One itch stopper doctors *don't* recommend is witch hazel, which most say will sting.

From the Inside Out

If topical measures fail you, most physicians say Benadryl is a good over-the-counter medication for itch. It is an antihistamine, which works by blocking the body's histamine chemicals that cause the itchy reaction to the virus. It also makes most people sleepy, so it's a good bet if your child is too itchy to sleep. As with all medications, you should carefully read the label and use the correct dosage for your child. Also remember not to use this medication along with a topical antihistamine (such as Caladryl), as this could cause an overdose.

POX IN UNPLEASANT PLACES

While some kids get through a case of chicken pox with just a few lesions on the torso, arms, and legs, others seem to get them everywhere. Pox can show up on the scalp, in the ears, in the mouth, or in the genital areas. The most troublesome of these tend to be those in the mouth and on the genitals. Sores in the mouth that break can make eating more difficult.

If your child has painful mouth sores, he should avoid acidic foods such as orange juice in favor of more gentle foods, like milk.

Usually children don't complain much about their mouth sores, but if they do, giving cold things to eat and drink can help numb the sores and make them less painful.

—DEAN BLUMBERG, M.D.,
UC DAVIS CHILDREN'S HOSPITAL

Genital lesions can make it uncomfortable to sit and urinate, and can be especially difficult to keep clean and dry.

Sitting in a cool bath can help ease the discomfort of lesions on the genitals, as can acetaminophen. Do your best to keep them clean and dry, and have your child wear loose clothes.

—BEN GITTERMAN, M.D.,
CHILDREN'S NATIONAL MEDICAL CENTER,
WASHINGTON, D.C.

If your child's lesions are so painful that she doesn't want to go to the bathroom, contact your pediatrician. Also be watchful for these "hidden" lesions, because they could get infected without your noticing.

Unfortunately, there isn't anything you can do about the number of pox your child has. Joseph Bocchini, M.D., of Louisiana State University Medical Center, says that talk about cool baths reducing the number of lesions, or warm baths causing a faster breakout but shortening the course of the illness, is just old wives' tales. According to Bocchini, the number of lesions a child gets is directly related to the "dose" or amount of virus present in the body; this is determined by the amount of virus he was exposed to and his own immune system.

FIGHTING FEVER

Doctors overwhelmingly recommend acetaminophen for treating the fever that accompanies chicken pox. While ibuprofen is also generally considered safe, because it is an immune system suppressant, some researchers had questioned whether it might raise the risk of secondary bacterial infection. A Boston University School of Medicine study published in the May 2001 issue of *Pediatrics* concluded that ibuprofen does not increase the risk of secondary infection, but if you have a choice, it is probably worth using acetaminophen instead. One thing research has proven is that children with chicken pox should not be given aspirin, which isn't as easy to avoid as you might think.

> Every time you give your child any medication, check the ingredient label first. You never know what has aspirin in it.
>
> —BEN GITTERMAN, M.D.,
> CHILDREN'S NATIONAL MEDICAL CENTER,
> WASHINGTON, D.C.

Giving aspirin to a child with chicken pox increases her risk of Reye's syndrome, a potentially fatal complication. Many cold remedies and other over-the-counter preparations do contain aspirin, including medicines for stomach upset, such as Pepto-Bismol. When you read the "active ingredients" section on the label, look for "salicylic acid." If you find it, avoid giving your child that product and find an aspirin-free alternative.

Doctors point out that treating a fever isn't always necessary. In fact, the fever is there to help fight off the infection itself. Unless your child has an *extremely high* fever (104 degrees Fahrenheit or above, the doctor may not suggest you treat it.

Reye's Syndrome

According to the National Reye's Syndrome Foundation, Reye's syndrome is a disease that impacts all the body's organs, with its most often fatal complications coming from its effect on the liver and the brain. It almost always follows some type of viral infection, such as a cold, the flu, or chicken pox.

Early symptoms include vomiting, lethargy, and unusual drowsiness. Later symptoms include irritability and unusually aggressive behavior, confusion, delirium, convulsions, and coma.

Symptoms of Reye's syndrome usually appear as the child is beginning to recover from the viral infection. If the disease isn't diagnosed and treated early, it can be fatal within days, so it is important to call your doctor immediately if your child has or has had a viral illness and develops these symptoms.

Aspirin has been associated with Reye's syndrome in children. It's a common ingredient in medicine, but not always a readily apparent one.

Common brand names for aspirin:
Bufferin
Bayer
Anacin
Ecotrin

Aspirin can also be found in many antacids, anti-nausea medications, arthritis medications, sinus medicines, and cough and cold preparations. Look for the words "aspirin" or "salicylate" on medication labels.

Other medications containing aspirin:
Alka-Seltzer
Alka-Seltzer Plus cough and cold medicine
Pepto-Bismol

Your child's level of activity, alertness, and responsiveness should help you decide whether to treat a fever.
> —MARK SCHLEISS,
> CHILDREN'S HOSPITAL
> MEDICAL CENTER OF CINCINNATI

If your child has a fever—even a relatively high one—but isn't acting particularly uncomfortable, it's okay to encourage rest and relaxation. On the other hand, if a child with even a low-grade fever is uncomfortable and lethargic, bringing the fever down can help her feel much better. Giving extra fluids is also important to prevent dehydration in kids with fever, and a cool drink can taste especially good to a child whose temperature is up.

WHEN TO CALL THE DOCTOR

In most people, chicken pox is a mild illness; younger children often have fewer symptoms and fewer lesions than older children or adults. However, the virus can cause some serious complications, including pneumonia, encephalitis (an inflammation of the brain), and serious bacterial infection of the lesions themselves. It can also evolve into a disease known as hemorrhagic chicken pox, which can be fatal.

> The great majority of chicken pox cases are mild, but parents need to be observant.
> —JOHN MODLIN, M.D.,
> CHILDREN'S HOSPITAL AT DARTMOUTH

Watch your child carefully during the illness, and contact your doctor if any of the following symptoms occur:

- If your child's lesions become especially red, swollen, or painful: This could be a sign of secondary bacterial infection
- If your child has fever beyond the third day of the illness: Again, this could be a sign of secondary infection
- If your child has exceptionally high fever (over 104°F)
- If your child is vomiting
- If your child shows signs of dehydration or pneumonia
- If your child is extremely ill or lethargic

If your child is lethargic, refusing to get out of bed, or falling down, see your doctor. This is a sign of cerebellar ataxia, a side effect that impacts coordination. It sometimes comes near the end of a course of chicken pox and generally resolves itself alone in a few days. It isn't generally serious, but it is worth having your doctor check it out.

—DEAN BLUMBERG, M.D.,
UC DAVIS CHILDREN'S HOSPITAL

- If your child's condition hasn't improved in three to six days
- If your child has what appears to be a relapse of illness once she has started to get better

Colic

You thought you brought a little angel home from the hospital. For the first week, you spent much of your time watching your new baby sleep peacefully and making glorious plans for the future. Now, however, it seems as if the baby hardly sleeps at all. Instead of watching over a sleeping angel, you find yourself bouncing, carrying, coaxing, and pleading with a little devil who just won't stop crying. You've tried everything you can think of—all the kind advice your friends and family could dish out—and now you're left facing the "C" word: colic.

Doctors can't explain colic, but they know it when they see it. And most do agree on a general definition. A colicky baby is otherwise healthy but has unexplained bouts of crying for more than three hours a day, at least three times a week, for at least three weeks in succession. Bouts of crying can happen at any time but are most common from five or six P.M. to midnight. They generally last at least forty-five minutes, and we're not talking about simple "fussing" here. A colicky baby screams at the top of his little lungs. The condition tends to show up by the time the baby is two or three weeks old and usually tapers off around six weeks, though for some unlucky parents it can last as long as six months.

Keep in mind that "normal" babies also exhibit this crying pattern to some extent (their crying peaks around six weeks, and crying is more common after five or six P.M.). It is helpful to know that babies have a range of crying that varies from quiet to excessive, and that parents have thresholds of tolerance that range from low to high. Sometimes what appears to be colic is just the unfortunate pairing of a baby who cries a lot but is normal with parents who have a low tolerance threshold.

Theories about what causes colic run the gamut from the stresses of everyday life on a baby's immature nervous system to unmet needs to food allergies to gas to anxious parents to bonding problems between parent and child. In the words of at least one doctor, the truth is that experts don't really know more about the cause than parents do. Just because we don't know what colic is, however, doesn't mean it's not real. It happens with at least one in every five babies.

One thing all doctors stress: Colic is *not* caused by bad parenting.

FIRST RESPONSE

CHECKING UP

The first natural step if your baby is having a crying jag is to make sure he doesn't need anything. Check the diapers, make sure he isn't hungry or too warm or cold, and see that he is otherwise comfortable. Also try to determine if he's tired, bored, or overstimulated. Don't be surprised if you don't find

What Colic Isn't

Though doctors either don't know or can't agree on what colic is, it's fairly easy to make a list of what they think it *isn't*.

A MILK ALLERGY

Though a small number of colicky children do have a milk allergy, those children generally have diarrhea and/or vomiting in addition to their colicky symptoms.

—Candice Johnson, M.D.

FORMULA INTOLERANCE

While symptoms might be similar, formula intolerance is not colic. Note that it can take as much as two to three weeks for an improvement once you've changed formulas. It takes that long for the old formula to get completely out of the baby's system.   —Michael Haight, M.D.

GASTROESOPHAGEAL REFLUX (GER)

This condition, in which the baby regurgitates much of what he eats, is sometimes mistaken for colic. Unlike colic, however, GER causes vomiting and poor weight gain.

—Michael Haight, M.D.

AN EAR INFECTION

Ear infections, like colic, cause unexplained bouts of crying. The difference is that symptoms of ear infection come on abruptly rather than gradually, and with ear infection, fever is generally present.   —Candice Johnson, M.D.

A TRAPPED HERNIA

Like an ear infection, this can cause unexplained crying. However, a colicky baby can eventually be comforted, or will stop crying on his own. An ill child will not.   —Cheryl Boyd, M.D.

anything wrong. In a colicky baby, a crying jag will often start for no reason at all, so don't feel guilty or go nuts wondering what you did to bring this on. Conversely, with a normal baby, you can usually tell what started the crying.

Check for any signs of illness. Colicky babies have a good sucking reflex and a healthy appetite. Colicky babies may spit up, but they don't vomit. True vomiting is a sign of some other problem.

If your baby routinely suffers from unexplained bouts of crying, and you are beginning to suspect colic, consult your pediatrician. The doctor should do a thorough medical exam to make sure there is nothing physically wrong with the baby. There are some medical problems that could look a lot like colic, especially in their early stages. These include hernia, a digestive disorder called gastroesophageal reflux (GER), heartburn, and ear infection. There are generally other symptoms associated with these medical conditions, and they do not come on gradually, as with colic. If you notice an acute change in your child's crying pattern, or symptoms such as vomiting, fever, or loss of appetite, see your doctor right away.

COMFORT CARE

Most of your initial efforts to address colic should focus on getting the help *you* need and having the right attitude toward the condition. After that, you can start to sort out coping strategies and a plan of attack. Above all, remember that colic isn't forever.

MOM AND DAD CARE

Take a Break

The first and perhaps most important thing to realize if you have a colicky baby is that your baby's condition is *not your fault.* Colic isn't the result of bad parenting, or a poor mother–child bond. Some doctors do claim that anxious parents can make the problem worse, but others say that it's the colicky baby who creates the anxious parents—not the other way around. Don't start feeling guilty because you aren't able to "fix" your baby's problem or because you're unhappy with the situation. Give yourself a break in every way possible.

> The biggest mistake parents make is blaming themselves for the colic and getting into a negative mindset. There is only so much the parents can do, and it is extremely important for them to have some time away from the baby. Find someone else who can take care of her for a night, a day, or even an hour.
>
> —CLIFFORD DAVID,
> WOLFSON CHILDREN'S HOSPITAL,
> JACKSONVILLE, FLORIDA

As exhausted as they are, some parents are reluctant to take the breaks they need because they feel no one else can care for the baby. However, if you don't take a breather, you'll quickly find that you don't have the energy to care for the baby, either. To make sure the break time isn't cut short, some doctors recommend that you have someone take the baby away from the house, rather than leaving the baby with someone at home. Worried parents will often rush back to check on the baby rather than get the rest they need. Also, parents of colicky babies are often too tired to get much enjoyment from going out; you can use the time alone at home to nap or relax.

Dear Diary

Keeping a colic diary is a good way for parents to keep track of what's happening with their baby, both for themselves and for their child's doctor. It's sometimes difficult for an exhausted parent to remember details about the last crying jag, or what might have worked to stop it. The diary keeps it all together and can give you a tool for strategizing. Record details of the baby's feedings, sleep, and crying episodes.

> Record what was going on when each crying period started, what you tried to do about it, and how long it lasted. This can help you spot patterns in your child's behavior and determine a strategy for dealing with it.
> —LESLIE FALL, M.D.,
> CHILDREN'S HOSPITAL AT DARTMOUTH

You can also use this diary to keep track of how your child's colic is progressing. Sometimes the intensity of a crying jag can make you forget that it's the baby's first one in two days, and that things are actually getting better. Using the diary to pinpoint your baby's "good" times of day allows you to use those times to plan for some pleasant bonding that will help you remember the good things about having a baby.

Many nursing mothers also use these diaries to record what they eat, since some doctors believe foods in the nursing mother's diet can contribute to colic in the baby. These "cryogenic" foods include all of the legumes (meaning beans of any kind) and other foods that produce large amounts of gas in the digestive system, says Michael Haight, M.D., of UC Davis Children's Hospital. Gas-producing foods include cabbage, Brussels sprouts, broccoli, asparagus, and other vegetables, and whole grains, according to the National Digestive Diseases Information Clearinghouse of the National Institutes of Health. Foods with lots of starch, such as potatoes, corn, and noodles, also might give you trouble.

Haight also recommends watching out for the "potential allergic type foods such as strawberries, nuts, dairy, and chocolate. Bland diets and avoiding sodas usually don't work very well," he continues.

If you are nursing and drinking large amounts of cow's milk, this might also give your baby trouble, says Candice Johnson, M.D., of The Children's Hospital, Denver. However, in this case your baby would have diarrhea, and possibly even bloody stools, which are symptoms of a food intolerance. Drinks high in caffeine, such as coffee, tea or tea drinks, and soda, can make your baby irritable and might contribute to colic, says Johnson.

Resetting Your Expectations

Pregnant moms are expecting in more ways than one. They expect a normal, healthy, happy baby. They expect cuddles and coos and smiles. They expect to have a relatively normal life, and even to be able to get a few things done while their little darling is napping in the afternoon. And they expect to adore just about every moment they spend with their new baby.

Parents with colicky babies have to let go of some of these expectations, at least for a while.

> Give up the idea of getting anything at all done while the baby sleeps. If your baby won't go down in her crib, get comfortable and hold and rock her while she sleeps. This will at least give you some peace and quiet and a bit of a mental break. You can read, watch television, talk on the phone, or maybe even nap with the baby. Just make sure you're in a position where you won't roll over on the baby or let her fall.
>
> —LESLIE FALL, M.D.,
> CHILDREN'S HOSPITAL AT DARTMOUTH

If your child does happen to fall asleep, Cheryl Boyd, M.D., of the Children's Hospital of Illinois cautions against letting her take more than a three-hour nap during the day. Colicky or not, a baby who sleeps all afternoon won't want to go to sleep at night. Doctors also recommend accepting any help you are offered and taking full advantage of the generosity of family and friends. This includes both parents doing all they can to help and support each other.

> Parents come in pairs for a reason. Tag-team the child, handing him off between you and keeping in mind that both the baby and the parents will survive this.
> —ERIC SINGER, M.D.,
>   CLEVELAND CLINIC CHILDREN'S HOSPITAL
>   FOR REHABILITATION, CLEVELAND, OHIO

There will be times when, no matter what you try, your baby will not stop crying. These times can be the most frustrating and dangerous. If you ever feel yourself getting so upset that you worry about what you might do, doctors say that it is perfectly fine to put the baby safely in her crib and walk away. Take a shower, read, or watch TV for fifteen or twenty minutes, or call your spouse or a friend who can lend support. To help you get through this time, imagine your life six or eight months down the road, when the colic is over. Colic is physiology, not personality, and your baby's temperament and your life will have changed quite a bit in a year.

> If you suspect your stress may be contributing to your baby's colic, see your own doctor.
> —MICHAEL HAIGHT, M.D.,
>   UC DAVIS CHILDREN'S HOSPITAL

Doctors generally agree that colic doesn't run in families, and it hasn't been proven hereditary in any way. So don't let the fact that you battled your way through one child's colicky infancy stop you from having another. Your next child might show no signs of colic at all.

COLIC CARE

Walking and Rocking

Colicky babies like rhythm. Walking, rocking, and car and stroller rides, because of their gentle and repetitive motion, are some of the most common suggestions from doctors and mothers who've been there. Of course, not all these solutions are practical all the time.

> Do not drive your baby around in the middle of the night. Parents who haven't had enough sleep shouldn't be behind the wheel.
>
> —ERIC SINGER, M.D.,
> CLEVELAND CLINIC CHILDREN'S HOSPITAL
> FOR REHABILITATION

Thankfully, there are alternatives for when a drive or stroll around the block isn't practical. Since it seems to be the motion and vibration that calms the baby, look for things that will provide that continual motion. If you have money to spend, there are a few devices on the market that attach to the crib and provide both motion and white noise, similar to a car ride.

> Putting your baby in their car seat and putting the car seat on the dryer while the clothes are drying can have a calming effect. Just make sure you don't leave him there unattended, because the car seat and baby could be bumped off onto the floor.
>
> —JOHN P. PHILLIPS, M.D.,
> CARRIE TINGLEY HOSPITAL,
> ALBUQUERQUE, NEW MEXICO

Also try rocking in a chair, turning on the vacuum cleaner, or purchasing something that just makes white noise, such as a crib toy that plays human heart sounds. Try patting the baby's back and making "shushing" noises in a firm, monotonous rhythm. Try rattles; if one doesn't work or the baby grows accustomed to it, try another. A baby swing might also help, though you shouldn't use one until your baby can hold his head up, and you shouldn't leave him in it unattended.

When you do feel like getting out of the house—a good idea if you've been cooped up with a crying baby—a stroll might be just the thing. Sometimes that blast of fresh air is enough of a surprise to startle a baby out of a crying jag. If Mom has been dealing with the crying baby, Dad can head out the door with the front pack to give her a break, and vice versa.

> Put the baby's feet through the bottom of the Snugli and cross her arms across her chest before cinching the sides up securely. This technique feels awkward at first and takes some practice. Walk outdoors at a brisk pace (as if you were in a hurry) for around fifteen minutes to give the baby a chance to calm down. Do this when she is tired, and she should fall asleep.
>
> —LESLIE FALL, M.D.,
> CHILDREN'S HOSPITAL AT DARTMOUTH

One of Dr. Fall's favorite tricks is to use this technique at your local mall. Walk around the parking lot and outside the mall until the baby falls asleep. You can then go inside and shop, or even have something to eat, in peace and quiet. Getting out of the house this way can be reviving for Mom and Dad.

OTHER TIPS AND TRICKS

No one technique works all the time, or keeps working throughout the baby's colic. Burping in the middle of *and*

Babies and Gas

Many people think colicky babies cry because they have gas, mainly because of the way these babies behave. They stiffen up or double over while they cry, and sometimes a burp helps. Doctors are in agreement that colic is not gas, but that colicky babies obviously do have gas—because of all that air they swallow while they are crying. While relieving the gas won't resolve the colic, it can certainly help make your baby more comfortable.

It's the pressure gas exerts on the tummy that hurts. In addition to pumping the baby's legs, try putting him across your legs or over your shoulder so that the gentle pressure on the tummy will equalize the pressure inside. Do not put baby on his tummy to sleep, as this has been shown to increase the risk of sudden infant death syndrome (SIDS).

If you are bottle-feeding and your baby has gas, try collapsible-bag bottles, which minimize the amount of air your baby swallows. Frequent burping during feedings is also important to babies who get gas. Sometimes a baby will need to be burped after each ounce or two. Make sure you sit the baby upright, and be persistent. Many parents don't pat long enough. Burp the baby gently but firmly until you hear that little belch.

You can also try the "football hold," in which you lay the baby facedown along your arm, head supported by your hand. The pressure of your forearm can help ease the pressure of gas in the baby's belly.

after feeding can help dispel painful gas, as can gently "pumping" the baby's knees up to his chest while he's lying flat on his back—you may get a few "toots" out to ease the gas pressure.

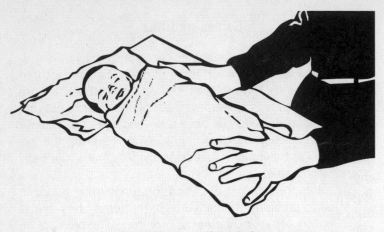

Swaddling a colicky baby.

Swaddling

Never underestimate the secure feeling of swaddling to calm a baby. Spread a baby blanket in a diamond shape on the ground. Fold the top tip down; this will go behind the baby's head. Place the baby face up in the center of the diamond, then fold the bottom tip up over the legs. Take the right side of the blanket and draw it snugly across the baby's chest, tucking it behind the baby's right shoulder. Then take the left side of the blanket and tuck it behind the left shoulder. You're aiming for a nicely tight bundling. Ask your doctor or nurse to watch your technique.

If you have tried to calm your baby without success for an hour, try this "last resort" remedy. Mix three ounces of very warm water with one ounce of apple juice, making the mixture as warm as you would a bottle. Give one ounce of this mixture to your baby. Don't use more than one ounce of this mixture more than once a day. It was often the only thing that worked on my daughter's colic.

—CHERYL BOYD, M.D.,
CHILDREN'S HOSPITAL OF ILLINOIS
AT OSF ST. FRANCIS MEDICAL CENTER

It's a good idea to discuss any herbal or home remedy that you are considering with your doctor first. Doctors recommend against giving more than four ounces per day of any herbal preparation or home remedy, even if they've approved it, and caution that some types of herbal preparations can contain ingredients that might harm your baby. Some parents have had luck with cooled chamomile tea, though doctors caution it should be made with bottled water and commercial tea bags, not home-grown plants or bulk herbs. Beware especially of anything containing belladonna, which is a strong narcotic. Doctors don't generally recommend over-the-counter medications that claim to be cures for colic, and some even caution against prescription medications. Others okay the use of anti-gas drops such as Mylicon; check with your pediatrician.

Most medicines for colic that actually work contain sedatives and antihistamines, which can have potentially dangerous side effects. Colic is not usually something you want to medicate.

—CLIFFORD DAVID, M.D.,
WOLFSON CHILDREN'S HOSPITAL,
JACKSONVILLE, FLORIDA

Some doctors say they will occasionally prescribe medications for colicky babies whose parents seem to have run out of patience and options. Generally, these prescriptions are designed to get the parents through until the colic resolves on its own. There is no actual "cure" for colic.

Overcoming Overstimulation

Doctors report that babies with colic seem more prone to overstimulation and are usually happier if they are handled gently and calmly. One theory says that this is because babies with colic simply have nervous systems that take longer than normal to mature, so are having trouble adjusting to the outside world. Overbouncing this baby or pacing restlessly can make the crying worse. One thing to try if your sensitive baby is beginning a colicky episode is to do nothing rather than something.

> Letting them try and cry it out for fifteen minutes won't hurt. If you are trying other calming techniques, don't switch techniques more often than every fifteen minutes. Use a timer to enforce this, because fifteen minutes can seem like forever when your baby is screaming at the top of her lungs.
>
> —CANDICE JOHNSON, M.D.,
> THE CHILDREN'S HOSPITAL, DENVER

Parents dealing with a colicky child might be tempted to try one thing after another if the first technique fails, but doctors say this can be just the type of overstimulation that upsets the child. Focus primarily on one calming technique—some doctors say for as long as three or four days—before switching to something else. If you're using the "cry it out" technique, first make sure the baby doesn't need anything—food, a diaper change, etc. Then put on some soft music or monotonous white noise, or make sure the room is quiet and dark.

Once they're in there, don't disturb them. Peek, but don't stimulate them more. Sometimes what you need is to do less and wait for it to go away.

—MICHAEL HAIGHT, M.D.,
UC DAVIS CHILDREN'S HOSPITAL

Even when they're not in the middle of a crying spell, colicky babies tend to get overstimulated easily. Be aware of noise, lights, and other stimuli in the house that might set your baby off. Because these children exist in a very high state of arousal, it is often difficult to calm them down enough to eat or sleep, even when they are hungry or tired.

WHEN TO CALL THE DOCTOR

It's a good idea to mention that you suspect colic to your doctor right away. You should also check back with your doctor if you don't feel the techniques you're trying are going well. Other reasons to call the doctor include:

- Acute changes in your child's crying patterns or pitch (the cry is suddenly very high and reedy, or barking) or other symptoms; colic comes on gradually, but radical changes in behavior usually indicate a medical condition
- If your child's symptoms appear *for the first time* when the baby is already two to four months old
- If nothing you try to calm your baby is working *at all*
- If your baby is having three or more episodes of colic a day
- If your baby's symptoms are not beginning to resolve by age four or five months

- If your baby has vomiting or diarrhea or is not gaining weight properly
- If your baby develops any other symptom not previously associated with the colic
- If you are ever uncertain about your child's condition, or if an episode of colic seems more severe than normal

Congestion and Stuffy Nose

Sneezing, dripping, stuffed-up noses are signs of the most common illness in children—the cold. Doctors say to expect six to eight of these upper respiratory adventures a year, even in the healthiest children. Having up to twenty colds in a year is not that unusual for the average child; there are a hundred to two hundred different viruses that can cause them.

The congestion that comes along with them can make it difficult for babies to eat and make life miserable for older children. The worst part is that there's no cure. A treated cold lasts a week, and an untreated one seven days, which leaves parents to find a way to keep their child comfortable until the congestion clears up on its own. Another common cause of runny nose and congestion is allergies, which can be difficult to distinguish from a cold.

FIRST RESPONSE

SERIOUSLY STUFFY?

Runny nose and congestion occur when the sinus, trachea (windpipe), and breathing passages are weeping mucus because of an irritation (antigen). Damage caused by the antigen also makes the nasal passages swell, leaving even less space for breathing. Because this antigen can be an allergen, infection, or other irritant, colds are not the only causes of congestion. Your first concern should be determining whether the congestion comes from something more serious.

> Many children don't seem to mind a runny nose, but from a hygiene point of view, it can be highly infectious. Teach your children to blow and wipe their noses to prevent the spread of infection to others.
> —JAMES LABAGNARA, JR., M.D.,
> ST. JOSEPH'S CHILDREN'S HOSPITAL, NEW JERSEY

If your child is wheezing, flaring her nostrils when breathing, or showing other signs that she's having significant trouble breathing, check with your doctor right away. This could be a sign of asthma (see "Asthma") or some other serious illness.

If your younger child seems to have congestion or drainage from one nostril only, look to see if he has something lodged inside his nose. If so, you'll probably need to visit the doctor to have the item fished out.

You'll also need to figure out whether the congestion is in the nose or the chest.

Foreign Objects in the Nose

Many doctors have funny stories about the things they have fished out of young children's noses. But under some circumstances, it is anything but funny.

You're most likely to discover the object if your child's nose is running on one side but not the other. Even if you can clearly see the object, *do not try to remove it yourself*. You might just end up pushing it farther in. Because the nasal passages are connected to the trachea, the item could even end up in your child's lungs, so leave the nasal expeditions to the professionals.

You have special cause for concern if you suspect that the object in your child's nose is a watch battery. These small, disklike batteries fit easily into the nasal passages and are filled with material that can very easily erode the skin. The battery needs to be removed by a doctor as soon as possible.

A rattle in the chest does not necessarily mean congestion in the chest. It could be an echo from the nose. A gagging cough or wheezing are more reliable signs of chest congestion.

—MARTHA DEBOLT, M.D.,
NEMOURS CHILDREN'S CLINIC,
JACKSONVILLE, FLORIDA

Chest congestion is usually a sign of something more serious than the common cold, and is generally worth a call to the doctor.

Antibacterial Soap

There are currently more than 700 different types of household products on the market that contain antibacterial agents, according to Stuart B. Levy, M.D., of Tufts University School of Medicine. These, of course, include liquid soap for hands, but that might not make your hands any cleaner.

In a June 2001 conference presentation to the U.S. Centers for Disease Control and Prevention (CDC), Levy asserted that "[antibacterial agents] are now being added to products used in healthy households, even though an added health benefit has not been demonstrated."

Levy cited several studies that found bacteria resistant to triclosan, the antibacterial agent most often found in household antibacterial soaps. In one experiment, researchers found that to kill *E. coli* bacteria—often found in uncooked beef—required two hours of exposure to triclosan soap at a temperature of 98.6 degrees Fahrenheit. Mutant strains that had become resistant to triclosan required two to four times longer to kill. "Most important, the time, temperature, and amount needed to kill the bacteria greatly exceeded the average five-second handwashing performed by most people," Levy said.

In the March–April 2001 issue of the CDC publication *Emerging Infectious Diseases,* Elaine Larson, RN, Ph.D., of the Columbia University School of Nursing in New York writes that plain soap should suffice for routine washing for the general public. For those with an extra need to keep the hands bacteria-free—such as people in close contact with newborns, the immunosuppressed, people who are ill, or people who work in childcare centers or preschools—Larson says that alcohol hand rinses are more effective.

These, she says, are widely available over the counter, kill a wide range of bacteria, and don't pose the threat of developing resistant bacteria.

COMFORT CARE

Assuming you're just dealing with a common cold or other upper respiratory infection, you can move on making your child more comfortable while you both wait out the illness. Comfort care for a child with runny nose or congestion focuses on keeping the nasal secretions (known to us parents as "snot") thin enough to run easily out of the nose, and keeping the nose clear enough that your child can relax.

LIQUIDATION

Extra Fluids

One of the most important things doctors agree that you can do for a child suffering from chest congestion is to keep him well hydrated. This means giving him plenty of fluids. Because a child with a stuffy nose is forced to "mouth breathe," he is more susceptible to dehydration. And if your child has a fever (see "Fever") along with her cold, she is even more likely to dry out.

> When your child is congested, the cells in the nasal passages are also losing fluid. Replenish this lost fluid with Gatorade, Pedialyte, and other fluids, because fluids are the best decongestant known to man.
>
> —KEITH PERRIN, M.D.,
> CHILDREN'S HOSPITAL, NEW ORLEANS

Doctors say that except in cases of extreme dehydration (when electrolyte replacement solutions like Pedialyte are best), any type of fluid your child will take is fine. This includes ice pops and Jell-O.

Frequent trips to the bathroom (or frequent wet diapers for babies) should tell you your child is getting enough to drink.

Humidifying

Getting plenty of fluids hydrates your child from the inside; you can use a vaporizer or humidifier to hydrate the nose from the outside. This won't cure your child's cold, or even shorten its course, but it can make her feel more comfortable.

There are two types of humidifier; warm mist and cool mist. Doctors who recommend them generally prefer the cool-mist sort, because of the danger of burns if your child comes in contact with the warm–mist machine. Warm mist, however, doesn't need to be cleaned as often, since the heat kills bacteria that might grow in the water and spread into the room.

> If you cannot secure a warm-mist vaporizer so that you are certain your child will be safe from the risk of burns, use a cool-mist model instead. Clean these at least weekly during periods of heavy use. Cleaning the machine with undiluted white vinegar and then rinsing with water works reasonably well, but the best thing is to take the machine apart and wash everything with soap and water. Also remember to change the filter.
>
> —KEN WIBLE, M.D.,
> CHILDREN'S MERCY HOSPITAL,
> KANSAS CITY, MISSOURI

Bleach and water is another good way to clean the machine, and you should change the water daily as well. Vaporizers/humidifiers are said to be especially good in dry climates, where the air doesn't hold much moisture, and during the winter when home heating dries out the air.

> The packaging on vaporizers and humidifiers usually has recommendations about the size of the room they are designed to work in. Make sure you choose the correct size machine for your child's room. One that is

too small won't put enough moisture into the air to do
any good.

—Cynthia Ferrell, M.D.,
Doernbecher Children's Hospital,
Portland, Oregon

Most doctors advise against humidifiers if your child has
allergies or asthma. The extra moisture can lead to mold
growth in the child's room, which may cause problems if
your child is allergic or if this is one of their asthma triggers
(see "Asthma"). Doctors also remind parents that there is no
real medical reason to use a vaporizer. They are just there to
help your child feel more comfortable.

UNSTUFFING THE NOSE

Suction

For babies, staying hydrated to help ease congestion presents
a catch-22. If your baby's nose is stuffed, she won't be able to
nurse or take a bottle, because she won't be able to breathe
and drink at the same time. And if she can't take a bottle or
nurse, she will become dehydrated and congested.

Be especially careful to keep your infant's head elevated when feeding, and avoid bottle propping. It's also
a good idea to suction the nose before feeding. The
sucking action can draw fluid into the eustachian tubes
inside the ear and cause infection.

—Harvey Kagan, M.D.,
Children's Hospital of the King's Daughters,
Norfolk, Virginia

To clear the nose so that baby can eat, doctors recommend
using plain saline (salt and water) nose drops and a bulb syringe.

The drops help to soften and thin the mucus so that it can be cleared out more easily. Several types are available at grocery and drugstores, and many doctors say the spray variety is better than the drops, as it reaches more easily up into the nose.

> You can even make your own saline nose drops. Just dissolve half a teaspoon of salt in a glass of water. These can help clear mucus, but if your child resists too much, they aren't worth the effort.
>
> —JOEL SCHWAB, M.D.,
>   THE UNIVERSITY OF CHICAGO CHILDREN'S HOSPITAL

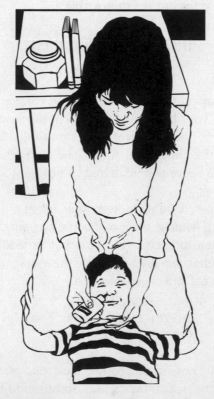

Holding your child's head to put in nose drops by yourself.

The best way to get the drops in is for your child to lie down, so the drops can work their way back into the nasal passages. Once the drops have had a few minutes to work, you can use a syringe to suction the nose, or have your child blow his nose if he is old enough.

> If you have to get saline drops into your child's nose by yourself, have her lie down and put her head between your thighs. Then tuck her hands gently under your legs so you can hold her still.
>
> —NESTOR VALERON, M.D.,
> MIAMI CHILDREN'S HOSPITAL

To properly suction the nose, get someone to help you hold the child's head still. A child who is young enough to need her nose suctioned (usually under age two) probably isn't old enough to understand what you are trying to do and is likely to put up some resistance. The tip of the syringe could injure her nasal passages if your child moves her head.

> Aspirators made to clear the ear actually work better for this than those made for the nose, because of the longer tip. Get a sturdy model with good suction, and be firm but careful. If the outside of the nostril becomes raw, you've overdone it. A little Neosporin can be used to soothe the skin.
>
> —KEITH PERRIN, M.D.,
> CHILDREN'S HOSPITAL, NEW ORLEANS

Once your child is still, squeeze all of the air out of the bulb while it's still *outside* your child's nose, then use the syringe to suction out as much mucus as you can. Again, be careful not to touch the tip of the syringe to the inside of your child's nose. Just go after what you can see, and don't use suction to clear really deep congestion.

Bulbs can also be sources of infection. Dispose of them after using during a child's illness, or at least make sure you clean them with *very* hot water before using them again.

—Cynthia Ferrell, M.D.,
Doernbecher Children's Hospital,
Portland, Oregon

Doctors recommend making this procedure as quick as possible (another good reason to have someone help you hold the child still), and to limit it to times when your child is feeling very uncomfortable, or when your baby needs her nose cleared so she can eat. Otherwise it isn't necessary and can even irritate the nose if overused. In fact, you shouldn't suction for more than three or four days in succession. Otherwise, you might actually make the problem worse.

Irrigating the nose with saline is a great way to clear up runny nose and stuffiness.

- For a baby or young child, use nasal saline drops that you can buy over-the-counter. Hold the child in a sitting position (maybe on the other parent's lap) and squeeze the saline gently into the nose, using a towel to catch the water that flows back out.
- For children over age six, fill a clean pot with warm water and a teaspoon or two of salt. Use a soft bulb syringe like you would use to suction an infant's nose. Have your child stand over the sink, fill the syringe with water, and squirt it into the nose, spitting out any water that flows into the mouth.

Do this a couple of times a day to keep the mucus washed out of the nose.

—Nina Shapiro, M.D., F.A.A.P.,
Mattel Children's Hospital at UCLA

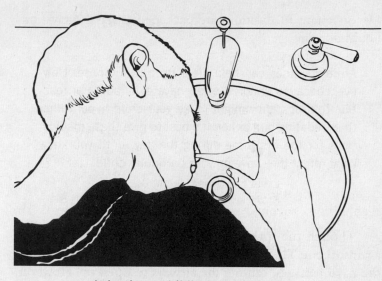

Irrigating a child's nose with saline.

Children can't blow their noses the same way adults do, blowing through both nostrils at once. To make it easier, teach your child to close one nostril and try to blow out of the other.

—HARVEY KAGAN, M.D.,
CHILDREN'S HOSPITAL OF THE KING'S DAUGHTERS,
NORFOLK, VIRGINIA

Medication

The "cold and flu" aisle of most supermarkets and drugstores is full of sprays and elixirs of every sort that promise to clear stuffy noses and stop the drips. There are more than a thousand over-the-counter cold preparations available, but these get mixed reviews at best from doctors, who say they often don't work and can have unpleasant or dangerous side effects.

Decongestant medications are packaged as nasal sprays, oral liquids, or pills.

> Antihistamines can help clear up a runny nose. However, because children often have a paradoxical reaction to drugs, they might make your child hyper rather than sedating him or her. It's best to give these medications for the first time during the day, until you know what effect they have on your particular child.
> —LAMES LaBAGNARA, JR., M.D.,
> ST. JOSEPH'S CHILDREN'S HOSPITAL, NEW JERSEY

Though the sprays are effective, doctors tend to advise against them. They work by constricting blood vessels inside the nasal passages, causing the airways to open up. However, the sprays themselves can eventually irritate the passages, which causes swelling and creates more congestion. Parents often combat this new congestion with more nasal spray, creating a vicious cycle known as the "rebound effect." Doctors note that because children's nasal passages are smaller than those of adults, they are more susceptible to rebound. In addition, these medications can sting; they don't help to shorten the course of the illness; and they could become addictive. At best, they should be used sparingly in cases of extreme congestion, for no more than two or three days at a time, in children twelve and older.

> If your child is in day care and has a chronic runny nose, you might want to try pulling him out for a week or two to see if that helps. You might also try to find a facility that groups fewer children together. Studies have shown that groups of ten or fewer kids are best.
> —NINA SHAPIRO, M.D., F.A.A.P.,
> MATTEL CHILDREN'S HOSPITAL AT UCLA

Doctors aren't quick to recommend oral decongestants and antihistamines, either; most find them ineffective, with potential side effects. Some doctors say they should never be used at all, while others say that they can have limited benefit but need to be used carefully and correctly. These medications tend to fall into three classes: decongestant, antihistamine, and combination products.

Decongestants (pseudophedrine found in brands like Sudafed, is a common type) work by drying up the nasal passages. Some doctors say that this just serves to make the secretions thicker and more difficult to clear, and ultimately makes the child more uncomfortable. Antihistamines are effective only if the congestion is caused by an allergy, rather than an upper respiratory infection; they work by blocking histamines, chemicals in the body that work to clear allergens from the body. They should never be given for a common cold. Combination medications might include doses of many different drugs, such as decongestant, antihistamine, cough suppressant, or fever reducer. Doctors say to avoid these entirely, because they often contain ingredients your child won't need for his specific symptoms.

> If you are going to use one of these medications, test it at home first on a day when your child isn't going to school to see how it affects her. That way you can avoid giving her something that makes her feel too drowsy or hyper and then sending her off to school.
>
> —CYNTHIA FERRELL, M.D.,
> DOERNBECHER CHILDREN'S HOSPITAL,
> PORTLAND, OREGON

Using any of these medications to clear congestion won't prevent your child's symptoms from progressing into an ear or sinus infection, according to doctors. These medications can also make your child feel either drowsy or hyperactive to the point where the side effects are more uncomfortable than the congestion itself.

Doctors specify that these medications should never be used in children under age five. If you do choose to use one in an older child, read the label, follow the dosing directions carefully, and call your doctor or pharmacist with any questions.

COMFORT ON THE NOSE

There are a number of other things you can do to make your child more comfortable until the illness runs its course.

Keep your child's head elevated, especially at night, to allow the secretions to run down out of the nasal passages rather than pooling in the nose or at the back of the throat.

> When elevating the head of a very young child or baby, place a pillow underneath the mattress or crib mattress rather than giving the child an extra pillow. Babies should never sleep with pillows, and with older kids, extra pillows slip out of place during the night.
>
> —MARTHA DeBOLT, M.D.,
> NEMOURS CHILDREN'S CLINIC,
> JACKSONVILLE, FLORIDA

This technique can also help to minimize swelling of the nasal passages. However, if the extra pillow or elevation makes your child uncomfortable, it's not worth using, since it's defeating the purpose.

To protect the nose and the delicate skin under it, make sure you have plenty of soft tissues on hand. There are even tissues treated with lotion available. Even the softest tissues, however, won't help if your child's skin becomes irritated: If

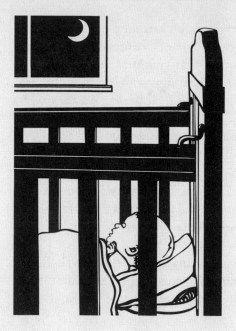

Placing a pillow under the crib mattress to elevate a baby's head.

it does, petroleum jelly or an antibiotic ointment will soothe. If your child is prone to licking his lips, K-Y jelly is a good choice.

> Rub a pretty-scented and flavored lip balm on the skin underneath your child's nose. Kids like the way it smells, and it can help keep the skin from getting irritated by the running and blowing.
>
> —Elizabeth Patrenos, M.D.,
> Children's Hospital at the
> Medical Center of Central Georgia

And what about the old standbys, chicken soup and vitamin C? Doctors say that both can be helpful, but mainly as a comfort rather than a cure. Chicken soup is a warm, steamy, tasty way to help get enough fluids into your child, and something about a hot bowl of chicken soup just makes a kid feel cared for. Though most doctors contend there are no studies to support the notion that vitamin C either prevents or shortens colds, many mention it as something with healing, anti-inflammatory properties. However, doctors warn against giving megadoses, saying that the amount in the typical multivitamin is enough. Overdosing can lead to ulcers, diarrhea, and other side effects.

The most important thing to remember is that none of these tactics are going to make your child get well more quickly. They are strictly to help your child feel more comfortable, so if they don't, there is no reason to use all or any of them.

> If your child is ill, the best thing you can do, if you can, is to take time out and stay home and be with him. If someone in your family is sick, respect that. Forget the schedule.
>
> —ELIZABETH PATRENOS, M.D.,
> CHILDREN'S HOSPITAL AT THE
> MEDICAL CENTER OF CENTRAL GEORGIA

WHEN TO CALL THE DOCTOR

When your child has a runny nose or is congested from a simple cold, you don't need to contact the doctor unless you suspect that something more than a cold is brewing. Signs that your child's cold is becoming a sinus or ear infection, or some other illness, are reasons to contact your pediatrician. These include:

- Your child has fever for more than three days, or poor color
- Your child has high fever or worsening cough

- Your child is having any trouble breathing
- Your child is not urinating as often as normal, or appears otherwise dehydrated
- Your child is irritable or lethargic
- Your child develops a rash
- Symptoms don't clear in seven to ten days
- Your child has a relapse of symptoms

Doctors say that the color of your child's mucus, contrary to popular belief, has little to do with whether or not your child has a sinus infection. According to Harvey Kagan, M.D., of Children's Hospital of the King's Daughters, the mucus is generally clear and watery during the first days of a cold. For the next two to three days, it will be thicker and often yellow or green. At three to five days, it will be even thicker and still often yellow or green; the white blood cells respond to the infection, and the body sheds them into the mucus. This is part of the normal progression of the cold.

If you have a baby or a very young toddler, especially one who is too stuffed up to eat, be especially vigilant. If your child has chronic congestion, the doctor will definitely need to evaluate it.

> If your child has chronic congestion, note what things seem to make him feel better—changes in environment, foods he eats or avoids—and report these to the doctor. This could help pinpoint the cause.
> —KEN WIBLE, M.D.,
> CHILDREN'S MERCY HOSPITAL,
> KANSAS CITY, MISSOURI

Most doctors do prefer to receive a call any time a parent suspects their child is "sicker than normal," or when the parent feels something is just not right. Even if your child isn't feeling especially ill, if her nose has been running for longer than two or three weeks, you should get your doctor to help you determine the cause.

If you do call, remember that there's a chance your doctor won't be able to do much to treat your child's cold. Unless she has a sinus or ear infection, or some other illness, antibiotics are useless, so don't demand them.

Conjunctivitis

Jeepers, creepers. The school sent your little one home with pinkeye? That's the more popular—and more descriptive—term for conjunctivitis, an infection or irritation of the conjunctiva membrane that makes up the underside of both the upper and lower eyelids. This unpleasant and unsightly, but rarely serious, condition comes in three forms: bacterial, viral, and allergic.

Bacterial conjunctivitis happens all year round and is most common in younger children. It is the result of a bacterial infection and causes a thick, green discharge that often "glues" the eyelid shut. To the child, it often feels like something is in the eye, but this type is not associated with much itching. "This is most common in the three-year-old range. Kids tend to get it in both eyes, along with an ear infection," says Raquel Martinez, M.D., of Miami Children's Hospital.

"It accounts for about eighty percent of conjunctivitis cases." When treated with antibiotics, bacterial conjunctivitis usually clears up in three or four days. Otherwise, it can drag on for as long as two weeks.

Viral conjunctivitis is associated with lots of itching and redness, but the discharge from the eye tends to be clear. It often comes at the same time as a runny nose or cough and is more common during cold and flu season in kids who are around eight years old. The duration of the infection depends on the specific virus involved, but can range from five days to two weeks.

Allergic conjunctivitis is not the result of an infection. Instead, the eye is irritated by an allergen of some sort. Its main symptoms are itching, redness, tearing and sensitivity to light, and a stringy white discharge. It is generally present in both eyes at the same time, and most often in children with a history of other allergic symptoms. It is more common in spring, summer, and fall.

FIRST RESPONSE

THE EYES THAT HAVE IT

The bacterial and viral forms of conjunctivitis are highly contagious, spreading from one person in the family to another in the blink of an eye, so to speak. The allergic form is not contagious, but since it is almost impossible for parents to tell which form their child has, your first course of action is to quarantine those red little eyes as much as possible.

It's important to wash hands frequently, both yours and your child's, to help control the spread of the infection. Your child should wash after touching her eye, and you should wash after cleaning or putting drops in her eye. Don't share towels and washcloths when cleaning up. Any towel or washcloth used on the infected eye, or by someone who has been tending to the infected eye, needs to be laundered in hot water. Keeping the eye itself clean is important, too.

> Keep the drainage clear from your child's eyes with a soft cotton ball or soft washcloth. This helps reduce the amount of infection present.
> —RANDALL KNOTT, M.D.,
> CARRIE TINGLEY HOSPITAL,
> ALBUQUERQUE, NEW MEXICO

Another vital step in controlling the spread of conjunctivitis is to get treatment from your pediatrician. Almost all cases of conjunctivitis will clear in about a week if left alone, but with treatment, the amount of time your child is contagious can often be shortened from ten days to one.

> If you can help it, don't clean out your child's eye until your doctor has seen it. Seeing the discharge will help her in diagnosing the cause of your child's conjunctivitis. If you need to clean the eye (if your child is upset because the discharge has sealed the eye shut), take a careful look at the discharge before you clear it away, so you can describe it to the doctor.
> —RAQUEL MARTINEZ, M.D.,
> MIAMI CHILDREN'S HOSPITAL

Only bacterial conjunctivitis responds to antibiotic treatment, but because it is difficult for even doctors to tell the differences among viral, bacterial, and allergic cases, they usually treat all conjunctivitis with antibiotics in drop or ointment form just in case. If your child's conjunctivitis is bacterial, it should clear within two or three days. Otherwise, it will likely take seven to ten days. In some cases, conjunctivitis is also associated with ear or sinus infections, and doctors generally check for and treat these things together. In rare cases, conjunctivitis can lead to a condition called orbital cellulitis, which means the infection has spread to other parts of the eye, so it's a good idea to see your doctor just to be safe.

Dropping In

Finding a treatment for conjunctivitis might be simple. Administering it is not. Trying to make a bull's-eye with that little drop of antibiotic or little line of ointment might seem harder with your squirming child than with the bull itself.

Most doctors will give you a choice of drops or ointment, and a number of factors come into play when making your decision. The first is whether or not you can get your child to hold still, or have someone to help you do so. Ointment tends to be more difficult to apply than drops, so choose drops if administering ointment seems completely unmanageable.

If your child is uncooperative, have him lie down on his back with closed eyes. Drip the eyedrop in the corner of the eye closest to the nose, then have him blink. The drop will roll right in.

—ANDREA B. LANIER, M.D.,
VALLEY CHILDREN'S HOSPITAL,
MADERA, CALIFORNIA

If your child is difficult but manageable, you might want to go with ointment. It doesn't generally need to be applied as often, so your struggle will at least be less frequent. Of course, children sometimes struggle because they know the medicine is going to sting. If this is the case, you have another reason to choose ointment, as it doesn't usually cause as much discomfort as drops. If you still want to use drops, there are some varieties that doctors say don't sting. Ask for one of these.

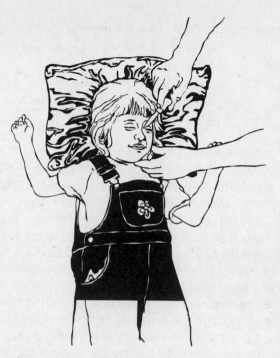

Putting an eye drop into the corner of a closed eye
so that it will roll into place.

Keep the eyedrops in the refrigerator. They won't
sting as much if they are cold, and it will help relieve
itching.

—RAQUEL MARTINEZ, M.D.,
MIAMI CHILDREN'S HOSPITAL

Nothing you choose will do much good if you can't get it
into the eye. Hygiene is important here, both to keep the eye
from being exposed to harmful bacteria and to help prevent
the spread of the highly contagious virus or bacteria that is
likely in your child's eye. So wash your hands and clean the
area around the eye.   (continued)

> Before putting in eyedrops or ointment, wet a wash-
> cloth with warm water and gently clear away any dis-
> charge around the eye.
>
> —Mohammed Jafar,
> Children's National Medical Center,
> Washington, D.C.

Throughout the process, don't touch the tip of the dropper or ointment tube with your hands, or against your child's
eye or eyelid. This will contaminate the dropper. It could also
injure your child's eye, which is an important reason to keep
your child as still as possible while you administer the drops
or ointment. If you can't get someone to help you with this,
try sitting on the floor and having your child lie down with her
head between your knees. You can tuck her hands gently
under your legs for added assurance.

When putting in drops, either have your child look up at
the dropper (so that the eye stays open) or hold his eyelids
open with your thumb and forefinger. Drop the dose in at the
side of the eye closest to the bridge of the nose. Another
option is to just hold down the lower eyelid and put the drop
in the pocket between the lid and the eye.

When using ointment, you'll need to hold your child
still and pull the lower lid down, then squeeze about a half-
inch line of ointment between the lids or in the lower eyelid
pocket.

> Squeeze ointment slowly, to keep the line of oint-
> ment from curling up against the end of the tube.
>
> —W. Scott Colliton, M.D.,
> Children's Mercy Hospital, Kansas

Doctors point out that a half-inch line of ointment isn't very
much, and that it isn't necessary to get a lot into the eye for
it to do the job. Less is better, as the ointment tends to be
messy.

It is best to use ointment just before putting your child to bed, so he doesn't have to be bothered if the medication's thickness temporarily blurs his vision.

—RAQUEL MARTINEZ, M.D.,
MIAMI CHILDREN'S HOSPITAL

Whether you're using ointment or drops, don't stop giving them before you've used the full course of medication prescribed by your pediatrician. Symptoms might clear up before treatment is finished, but that doesn't mean all the bacteria are gone. Stopping too soon could set your child up for a relapse.

COMFORT CARE

While you're waiting out your child's case of conjunctivitis—and it could be a long wait if that case is viral or allergic—focus on keeping the eyes clear and comfortable, minimizing itching, and easing any pain that might occur.

KEEPING A CLEAR EYE

If your child has conjunctivitis, especially bacterial, don't be surprised if he wakes up with his eyes "glued" shut with crusty discharge. This can be especially upsetting to younger children and babies, so you'll want to clear it fairly quickly. Once you have your child calmed down a bit, your best ally is water, to soften the discharge so the eye can open.

Irrigate the eye with preservative-free saline to take away the crust and get the eye to open.

—ANDREA B. LANIER, M.D.,
VALLEY CHILDREN'S HOSPITAL,
MADERA, CALIFORNIA

You can also try wetting the eye down with a clean washcloth, gauze, or cotton balls soaked in water. Never force the eye open, even to put drops in. If you absolutely cannot get the crust to soften, call your doctor rather than continuing the struggle and upsetting your child. Once you do manage to get the eye open, clean the crust away.

> Use a clean washcloth and no soap to wash away the discharge. Q-tips can help with the corners.
>
> —W. Scott Colliton, M.D.,
> Children's Mercy Hospital, Kansas

Use warm or cool water, whichever your child finds most comfortable. If her eyes are itching, cool water is often more helpful. When you are finished, dispose of used cotton or gauze, launder washcloths and towels, and wash your hands and your child's.

Along with the discomfort from the discharge, your child might experience mild pain caused by the swelling of the irritated membranes. Doctors say that acetaminophen (Tylenol) or ibuprofen (Advil) will usually relieve both swelling and pain; they cannot, however, remove the sensitivity to light that comes with some cases of conjunctivitis.

> If your child's eyes become sensitive to light, keep lights low and use sunglasses and hats to shade the eyes when going outdoors.
>
> —Mohammed Jafar, M.D.,
> Children's National Medical Center,
> Washington, D.C.

ITCHIES

Besides the redness, itching is one of the more annoying symptoms of conjunctivitis. In bacterial cases, it should start to subside within twenty-four hours of starting treatment, as the antibiotic begins to fight the infection. In allergic and viral cases, you will have a bit more of a wait: Doctors recommend cold compresses as a good way to treat itching and provide comfort.

> Have your child lie down and relax, and don't let her fiddle with the compress while it is on. Put on some music she likes to help distract her.
> —Andrea B. Lanier, M.D.,
>   Valley Children's Hospital,
>   Madera, California

In cases of allergic conjunctivitis, some over-the-counter antihistamine eyedrops can help decrease inflammation and itching, but it's best to consult your pediatrician about these. Some doctors warn that your child might not like them.

> Over-the-counter eyedrops can sting, they often dilate the pupil, and some have preservatives that some people are allergic to. Kids don't like them, and I don't think parents should use them.
> —Andrea B. Lanier, M.D.,
>   Valley Children's Hospital,
>   Madera, California

If you do try them with your doctor's blessing and they don't begin to work within three days, you should check back with your doctor before continuing to use them. An over-the-counter oral antihistamine such as Benadryl can be helpful and has the added benefit of making your child too drowsy to notice the itching. But these, too, should be used only with your doctor's approval.

WHEN TO CALL THE DOCTOR

Any child with conjunctivitis should already be under a doctor's care. During treatment, it's your job to watch for signs that the conjunctivitis has turned into something more complicated, or moved into another part of the eye. If your child develops the more serious infection called orbital cellulitis, treatment requires hospitalization and antibiotics. You might suspect complications if:

- Discharge increases instead of decreasing within two days of starting treatment
- Eyelids begin to swell or if your child cannot open her eyes
- Your child develops a fever
- Your child experiences changes in mood or behavior
- Your child's sensitivity to light increases
- Your child experiences severe or increasing pain
- There are changes in your child's vision or in the color of the eye
- There are visible defects on the surface of the eye

Newborns often have symptoms because of a blocked tear duct, which could become infected. If your newborn has eye problems, consult your doctor promptly.

—RANDALL KNOTT, M.D.,
CARRIE TINGLEY HOSPITAL,
ALBUQUERQUE, NEW MEXICO

You should of course call your doctor anytime you think something isn't going as it should. If symptoms persist for more than a week, your child should also be evaluated by an ophthalmologist. And if your child's allergic conjunctivitis is severe and recurring, the underlying allergy may need treatment before the problem will go away completely.

Constipation

If you've made it through potty training, it might seem like it took your child forever to learn when *not* to go. If you're still changing diapers, it can feel like your child goes constantly. Either way, you'll eventually run into a time when your child isn't going like he should. And when things grind to a halt like that, sorting out the problem can be tough.

FIRST RESPONSE

IS IT REALLY CONSTIPATION?

The answer to this question is "not necessarily." Just because your child didn't have a bowel movement today doesn't mean he's constipated. Doctors agree that the number of times per day isn't what counts so much as what is normal for your child. In fact, the normal range is anywhere from one bowel movement every three days to three bowel movements a day. Being familiar with the signs of constipation and with what is normal for your child is the only way to spot it.

Constipation in a child can be different than in an adult, so the classic signs—infrequent, hard stools that are difficult to pass—are not the only ones you might find. Other clues that your child is constipated include stomachache (especially one that goes away right after a bowel movement), blood in or on the stool or in the underpants, straining or pain during toileting, and stools so large they clog the toilet. Kids who are constipated might also lose their appetite and generally just not feel well.

One sign parents often miss is what appears to be diarrhea, or leaking of stool in the underpants. Called encopresis, this condition is most common in kids ages two to seven and occurs when a large, hard stool is impacted in the bowels and other stool leaks around it.

If your child is constipated, you'll need to find out what is causing the problem. If she is truly uncomfortable, you may have to soften the stools with medication to make them easier to pass.

COMFORT CARE

There is little you can do to comfort a child who is straining through a painful bowel movement, or is miserable because she cannot go. You should focus on solving the problem at hand, so that your child's constipation will go away and she can feel better. Low fluid intake, improper diet, and low activity level can all contribute to constipation. Big stresses and transitions—especially potty training—can also be factors.

To solve the underlying problem, look for any situations that might be causing your child stress. Also consider how physically active she is. Encouraging regular exercise is healthy for any child. In addition, consider her diet and bowel habits to identify things you can do to improve the situation.

FLUIDS

Make sure your child gets enough to drink, which helps the fiber you eat do its job, and keeps stools softer and easier to pass. This might be easier said than done. Children ages two to five need twenty-four to thirty-two ounces of water daily, according to Deise Granando-Villar, M.D., F.A.A.P., of Miami Children's Hospital. Older kids need even more, but most are too busy to sit down and drink that much.

> Buy a water bottle and keep it in the refrigerator to encourage water drinking.
> —JILL REEL, M.D.,
>   BOYS TOWN NATIONAL RESEARCH HOSPITAL,
>   OMAHA, NEBRASKA

Water and hundred-percent fruit juice are the best ways to keep your child hydrated, say doctors. Be sure you give plenty to drink with meals, since that's one time your child is almost guaranteed to be sitting still. Also provide water to drink away from home. Since it's common for people to carry around water bottles these days, this shouldn't cause your child embarrassment. You can even get reusable bottles with cartoon characters or sports logos on them.

> Send a water bottle to school so your child gets enough to drink throughout the day. Even if your child's school

doesn't normally allow them, few teachers will refuse if you tell them it's because your child is constipated.

—BARBARA FELT, M.D.,
MOTT CHILDREN'S HOSPITAL AT THE
UNIVERSITY OF MICHIGAN

Hikes, trips to the park, and sports practice are all good times to send along a bottle of cold water. If your child is in the habit of having it available, she'll be more likely to drink it.

DIET

What your child eats is important as well. Often changing the diet is the only way to resolve the problem of constipation. There are two factors here: what your child does and doesn't eat.

Fiber

One thing most kids *don't* like to eat is fiber—or rather, foods high in fiber. Doctors report that fruits, vegetables, and whole-grain breads and cereals are sadly lacking in the diets of most kids they see. Of course, parents often don't eat enough of these foods, either, and that's a good place to start. Try to have plenty of high-fiber healthy foods available for the whole family.

Go about this gently and make simple changes, such as using wheat instead of white bread, choosing a higher fiber cereal, or mixing some high-fiber cereal in with a kind your family likes. Read labels carefully if you want to do any good here. There are foods on the shelf that look and sound like they should have lots of fiber but really don't.

Fiber Facts

One of the main measures doctors recommend for preventing constipation is to get enough fiber into your child's diet. According to the American Dietetic Association (ADA), that means using the "age + 5" formula. Under this rule, a child who is eight needs thirteen grams of fiber a day, and a child of four needs nine grams.

Doctors recommend subtle dietary changes, rather than a big overhaul, to increase fiber intake. The ADA proposes several things you can do to increase fiber for the whole family.

Have high-fiber foods such as popcorn, nuts, fresh fruit, and raw vegetables ready for snack time. Breakfast is also a good time to find fiber; many breakfast cereals and breads are good sources. Check cereal labels to find one with five or more grams of fiber per serving, and choose whole-grain breads and muffins.

If your child likes legumes (beans), serve them two or three times a week to benefit from their excellent fiber content. You should also try to work at least five servings of fruits and vegetables a day into your family's diet, preferably with the edible skin on, which can add as much as a gram of fiber to foods like potatoes. When shopping, make a habit of reading food labels for the fiber content and fiber-adding ingredients such as bran or whole-grain.

By making a few of these simple changes and paying attention to your family's fiber intake, you can really make those grams add up.

Changing the diet of a child can be very difficult if you go about it radically. Instead, look at what she eats and focus on the foods that have more fiber. Encourage those but don't force them.

—GARY SILBER, M.D.,
PHOENIX CHILDREN'S HOSPITAL

You can also encourage foods like popcorn, or even try tricks like sprinkling bran or ground-up high-fiber cereal on foods your child likes. If you go the fruits-and-vegetables route, you know the fiber's there; it's just sometimes more difficult to get kids to eat them. Fruits are usually more appealing to children because they are naturally sweet. Most of the insoluble fiber that can speed stool through the bowels is in the peels of fruit and vegetables, so feed your child apple slices instead of applesauce, or baked-potato wedges instead of mashed potatoes. And a bit of creativity helps. You can hide fresh fruit under your child's favorite yogurt and call it a sundae. Or you can give dried fruit with pretzels or high-fiber cereal as a snack.

> If your child is not a big fruit eater, try mixing it with gelatin or marshmallows. You can also mix prune juice with soda pop to get them to drink it.
>
> —JILL REEL, M.D.;
> BOYS TOWN NATIONAL RESEARCH HOSPITAL,
> OMAHA, NEBRASKA

There may be times when you just have to be firm. Put a selection of healthy foods out there, and let your child choose among them. But don't give him the option of having something he likes better but really shouldn't eat.

> Parents sometimes let kids fill up on milk and sometimes don't make other healthy foods appealing to them. Parents also give up too easy when trying to get their kids to eat right. By the fourth, fifth, or sixth time you offer a food, they will likely eat it.
>
> —APRIL DOUGLASS-BRIGHT, M.D.,
> CHILDREN'S REGIONAL HOSPITAL AT
> COOPER, NEW JERSEY

If your child is old enough, talk to him about why fiber is important and how he can get more of it into his diet. Teach him about foods that are high in fiber, take him grocery shopping with you, and have him help choose the high-fiber foods he wants. At any age, children who are increasing their fiber intake must also make sure they get plenty of water. The water will make the stools softer and easier to pass.

Dairy

Doctors seem to have mixed feelings about dairy in the diet. On the one hand, it's an excellent source of the calcium kids need. On the other, the protein content in dairy can cause constipation. Most doctors advise that you back off dairy but don't eliminate it completely.

> Don't restrict dairy foods. Instead, encourage your child to eat plenty of other foods so that the amount of dairy she eats is reduced naturally. Cheese is one of most toddlers' favorite foods. If you eliminate that, you don't leave much they will want to eat, and it becomes a struggle.
>
> —JOE CLARK, M.D.,
> MEDICAL COLLEGE OF GEORGIA

You can also take a short break from dairy foods, then reintroduce them into your child's diet as the constipation starts to improve. Be aware that it's not just milk we're talking about here. For older kids, pizza—with its abundance of cheese—is a big culprit.

If your child is six to twelve months old, has just changed from formula or breast milk to cow's milk, and has become constipated, the best thing to do is switch him back to formula or breast milk. However, don't switch your baby to low-iron formula because of constipation. No study has proven that the level of iron found in infant formula is constipating.

Anemia, on the other hand, is a major concern, and the iron in formula helps to prevent it (see "Anemia"). Doctors do recommend that you avoid giving over-the-counter vitamins with extra iron to your older child if he's constipated.

Other Crumbs of Information

Dairy foods aren't the only ones that can constipate. Rice and rice cereals, bananas, and high-protein foods like meats can also contribute to the problem. Watch out for crackers and junk food—they fill kids up and they're low in fiber. High-caffeine foods such as tea, soda, and chocolate can also work against you. The best way to battle these is just to have less of them around the house. To get your kids to eat right, you have to eat right yourself.

Another part of eating right is *when* and *how* you eat. Running out to grab meals at fast-food restaurants limits your control over the foods your children choose, hampering your ability to provide a high-fiber diet.

> Eat on schedule. Try to avoid "on the go" meals where you have less control over what foods your kids are choosing. This also helps create a regular toileting schedule.
>
> —DEISE GRANADO-VILLAR, M.D., F.A.A.P.,
> MIAMI CHILDREN'S HOSPITAL

BOWEL HABITS

Your child's bowel habits start to form the day potty training begins. Unfortunately, most parents concentrate on the idea of teaching the child to "hold it" until she gets to the bathroom, but do little to establish a good toilet routine that encourages the child to go on a regular basis.

Put your child on a routine. After you eat, have her go to
the bathroom within half an hour. Try to destress it,
though, and don't have her sit for more than five minutes
if she doesn't want to. To motivate her try a star chart,
where she gets a star every time she goes.

—MICHAEL HAIGHT, M.D.,
UC DAVIS CHILDREN'S HOSPITAL

Some kids—especially those between ages two and five—
will just ignore the urge to go because they don't want to
interrupt their play, their television show, their video game,
or whatever else they're doing. This makes the muscles
tighten, while the stool gets harder and drier and eventually
becomes very difficult to pass. Eventually, they hold back
because it hurts to go.

You want to make sure your child tries to defecate at least
three times a day, if not more. This doesn't mean he needs to
have a bowel movement every time he sits, so don't pressure
him. And don't keep him there for a long time. Just make him
comfortable and let nature take its course. Don't let him
think he's being punished.

When having your child sit on the toilet, put a timer
there so that he can see how long he has to be there.

—GARY SILBER, M.D.,
PHOENIX CHILDREN'S HOSPITAL

To make this happen, regular toilet access is a must. That
probably won't be a problem at home, but school might be
another matter. Doctors report that many children develop constipation after beginning school because they don't want to use
the bathrooms there. Some schools have removed the stall
doors for safety reasons, and some school bathrooms are just plain
unpleasant to go into. There might also be a group of kids who
hang out in the bathroom and make your child afraid to go in.

Find out whether the bathrooms at school have doors. You can request that a child have access to a private bathroom (most schools have one reserved for the teachers) if necessary. You should also think about your child's schedule. Does she have time to go, especially after lunch? Arrange a time for her if necessary.

—BARBARA FELT, M.D.,
MOTT CHILDREN'S HOSPITAL AT THE
UNIVERSITY OF MICHIGAN

Another issue is that school lunches, recesses, and breaks between classes tend to be short, and kids often don't get enough time to go to the bathroom. But resisting the urge to go only makes the problem worse. If you explain the situation, your child's teacher or principal will probably be willing to help you arrange things so that she has a clean restroom to visit and a sufficient amount of time in which to go.

USE OF MEDICATIONS

If you've tried for a week or two to resolve your child's constipation through increasing fluids, eating properly, and encouraging good toilet habits and haven't had success, some form of medication might be necessary. There are three over-the-counter options for treating constipation, but they are best used under a doctor's care. Any of these options—laxatives, enemas, or glycerine suppositories—might be fine for one acute incidence of constipation, but they can have serious consequences if used incorrectly for chronic cases.

Laxatives

Doctors note some confusion over the meaning of the term "laxative," which actually means a drug that stimulates evacuation of the bowels. These should not be confused with "stool softeners," which do just what the name implies. Many doctors urge parents to stay away from bowel stimulants completely, because they can cause cramping and kids can become dependent on them if they're overused.

It is, doctors say, difficult for parents to tell whether the various over-the-counter products on the market contain stimulants. Even some "natural" laxatives made for children contain them. That's just one more reason to talk to your doctor first. Sometimes a product with stimulants might be necessary, but professional guidance is important. Your child's doctor can set up a treatment plan that keeps you from making two common mistakes: The first is giving laxatives for too long a period of time, which can make your child dependent on them for every bowel movement. The second is stopping treatment too soon, before the child's rectum—which is stretched from holding all that extra stool—is completely back in shape and ready to pass stool normally.

Common Stimulant Ingredients in Laxatives
- Bisacodyl (bis-a-KOE-dill)
- Casanthranol (cas-SAN-thrah-nole)
- Cascara Sagrada (kas-KAR-a sa-GRA-da)
- Cascara Sagrada and Aloe (kas-KAR-a sa-GRA-da and AL-owe)
- Cascara Sagrada and Phenolphthalein (kas-KAR-a sa-GRA-da and fee-nole-THAY-leen)
- Castor Oil (KAS-tor)
- Dehydrocholic Acid (dee-hye-droe-KOE-lik acid)
- Phenolphthalein (fee-nole-THAY-leen)
- Phenolphthalein and Senna (fee-nole-THAY-leen and SEN-na)
- Senna (SEN-na)
- Sennosides (SEN-no-sides)

There are two remedies many of our mothers likely associated with relieving constipation: castor oil and mineral oil. Both have been used for generations and are effective, but doctors offer the same cautions as with other preparations. Most caution against use of castor oil completely, because it's a stimulant; and they say that if you're planning to use mineral oil, you should check with your pediatrician first. The usual beginning dose of mineral oil is one tablespoon.

> Don't give your child mineral oil if she struggles to drink it. If she inhales it into her lungs, it could cause pneumonia. It shouldn't be used at all in children under a year old for this reason.
>
> —GARY SILBER, M.D.,
> PHOENIX CHILDREN'S HOSPITAL

Doctors once thought that mineral oil carried fat-soluble vitamins (like the B-complex) out of the body with it, thus preventing digestion and absorption of the vitamins. Many doctors have changed their thinking on this, but there is still some debate. For this reason, some doctors recommend that you wait to give mineral oil until after your child's food is digested.

> Mineral oil is reasonably safe but should be given away from mealtime, and never if your child is vomiting, because of the danger that he will inhale it. Don't use it regularly, however, unless you are consulting your doctor.
>
> —JOE CLARK, M.D.,
> MEDICAL COLLEGE OF GEORGIA

The mineral oil acts as a stool softener and lubricant, making the stools easier to pass. As with all medications, it is important to use as directed by the packaging or your pediatrician. Doctors also caution parents against giving your child any product meant for adults, and they say that you should not use any type of laxative product for more than a week without talking to a pediatrician.

Enemas

Enemas are another effective over-the-counter treatment for constipation. Preparations designed for use with children are readily available, and some doctors claim that giving one is no more complicated than taking a rectal temperature. However, an enema can have side effects or be uncomfortable if used incorrectly, so it's worth consulting your pediatrician if you've never given one before.

> Enemas can be traumatic for a child and can make constipation and toileting more of an issue than it already is. And if you give too much enema, you can cause an electrolyte disturbance, excessive loss of fluids, or abdominal cramping. Don't give your child an enema without consulting your doctor.
> —APRIL DOUGLASS-BRIGHT, M.D.,
> CHILDREN'S REGIONAL HOSPITAL AT
> COOPER, NEW JERSEY

In either case, never give a tap-water enema, as these can leach the sodium from your child's body and actually cause seizures. Everyone's body requires a certain level of sodium and electrolytes, which aren't contained in plain water. Too much plain water—either by mouth (if someone isn't eating) or in an enema—without added electrolytes can throw the body out of balance.

> Enemas are especially helpful in cases of encopresis, and are best given in the evening or on a weekend, so

the child has time to relax and free access to the toilet afterward. Parent attitude is very important when giving an enema. Be matter-of-fact but comforting. Explain why the enema is necessary, and that it will make things better.

—JILL REEL, M.D.,
BOYS TOWN NATIONAL RESEARCH HOSPITAL,
OMAHA, NEBRASKA

ATTITUDE

Your attitude is important in helping your child deal with constipation, especially if the constipation occurs when you're in the middle of potty training or if your child experiences fecal soiling.

If your child has been resistant to potty training, or if his constipation problems begin during the process, many doctors recommend you relax your expectations, at least until the constipation is resolved. This age is a difficult one for children, and the idea of potty training often clashes with the child's emerging sense of independence.

The right attitude is also vital if your child is past potty-training age and is experiencing fecal soiling. Parents sometimes mistakenly blame their child for soiling. This negativity can impact your child's self-esteem and behavior, so you need to remember that soiling is not your child's fault. You shouldn't be battling against your child, but working with her to solve the problem.

Call the doctor immediately if your child is soiling to get the education you need so you can have the right attitude toward the problem. Parents need to convey the idea that parent and child need to work together, and that things won't get instantly better. Don't focus on soiling. Be supportive and understanding, and don't punish.

—Barbara Felt, M.D.,
Mott Children's Hospital at the
University of Michigan

Solving the problem now will help keep it from becoming a problem as an adult. Many adults who have constipation report having problems from the time they were children, probably because they never corrected the bad habits that began when they were kids.

It goes without saying that you need to be comforting when your child—especially one who is very young—is struggling with one of those painful BMs. If you have a toddler, it might be difficult for you to tell whether your child is straining to pass the stool or to hold it in. Toddlers who have had painful bowel movements often try not to go again for fear it will hurt.

You can't really reason with toddlers. You have to use mineral oil to get the stool so loose that it comes out anyway. After a month or so of loose stools, they will figure out that they can relax. Keep this up for the full month (under a doctor's care, of course) or the stool will get hard again, and you're right back where you started.

—Joe Clark, M.D.,
Medical College of Georgia

If your child is holding his body straight and stiff, rather than doubled over, he is likely working to keep the stool in rather than get it out. Again, this practice is most common in toddlers. Older kids can understand that they need to go or the problem will only get worse.

You can use calendars and stickers to encourage them, plus lots of reassurance and positive reinforcement. The book *Everyone Poops* and others like it can help. Warm baths and backrubs can also help with cramping.

—JILL REEL, M.D.,
   BOYS TOWN NATIONAL RESEARCH HOSPITAL,
   OMAHA, NEBRASKA

If your child is young enough to want you there, be calm and soothing. You can read a book or even play a game to help distract him. It also helps to explain that once he's through, he'll feel much better.

You can use breathing techniques to help them "blow away" the discomfort. Have them blow on a pinwheel or a feather when it hurts.

—BARBARA FELT, M.D.,
   MOTT CHILDREN'S HOSPITAL AT THE
   UNIVERSITY OF MICHIGAN

Many children are frightened by the loss of control: They can't make their body do what they want it to do. If you sense your child is feeling this way, it might help to talk about all the things she can do to help fix the problem—like eating right, exercising, and going to the bathroom regularly. Help her regain that sense of control, and she'll feel better.

Also make your child as comfortable as you can. Play her favorite music, or let her bring a stuffed animal into the bathroom if that helps. Make it as pleasant a place to be as you can.

If your child's feet don't reach the floor when she's sitting on the toilet, give her a footstool to put under them
to make her more comfortable.

—April Douglass-Bright, M.D.,
                Children's Regional Hospital at
                Cooper, New Jersey

Another way you can encourage your child is to make
sure he knows that this problem will take some time to solve,
but that it won't go on forever. Explain that he will eventually
be able to use the toilet without pain, and that it won't always
be such a big deal. Having this to look forward to might make
the treatment plan and lifestyle changes easier to endure.

WHEN TO CALL THE DOCTOR

IN BABIES

Newborns generally have their first bowel movement within
twenty-four to forty-eight hours of birth, often while they're
still in the hospital. If you and your baby are already home
and she hasn't started having bowel movements by the second
day, that's reason enough to call the doctor. It probably means
there's something awry with the digestive system. For the
same reason, it's a good idea to check with your doctor about
any case of constipation in a child younger than two months.

If your child is healthy and breast-fed, there is little
chance he'll be constipated during the first year of his life. If
he is, something might be wrong with the digestive tract; this
is another occasion to call the doctor.

IN OLDER KIDS

If a child is old enough to express it, his discomfort will likely
be the first sign that something might be wrong. Many doc-

tors say they should see a child who cries during a bowel movement, complaining of extreme pain or constant pain in the abdomen for more than two hours.

Also call the doctor if you see blood in the stool or signs that your child has anal fissures. These are small tears in the anal area, which can be quite painful. Other reasons to call include fever, vomiting, or a firm, extended abdomen.

OVER TIME

No case of constipation resolves in a day. However, if your child goes more than four days without any bowel movement at all, or the remedies you've tried aren't starting to improve things in a week or two, it's time to seek your doctor's help. Your child also needs medical attention if she is constipated long enough to be losing weight, if the constipation seems to keep coming back, or if your child is constipated enough to have soiling problems.

Enlist your doctor's aid if your child isn't going along with the treatment program, is refusing to make dietary changes, take medications, or sit on the toilet when necessary.

Cough

The main thing doctors seem to want to remind parents about cough is that, in and of itself, it isn't an illness that needs to be cured. In fact, cough is a protective mechanism that helps clear secretions and irritants from our airways. So when the body is coughing, that mechanism is doing its job. However, there are times when cough can be inconvenient— such as when it keeps your child and you awake all night— and times when too much coughing can be troublesome.

FIRST RESPONSE

COUGH DETECTIVE

The only way to effectively treat a cough, according to doctors, is to treat the underlying cause. So the first thing you need to do if your child is coughing is to try and find out why.

Choking

According to the American College of Emergency Physicians
(ACEP), nearly four thousand men, women, and children die
from accidental choking in the United States each year. It's
important to know what to do if your child is choking.

Most doctors and child-care experts recommend that you
supervise your very young child while he is eating. Take basic
baby-proofing measures to make sure small objects are kept
out of reach.

> Children under the age of six should not be given
> nuts, hard candies, or even hot dogs to eat because
> they can choke on them. If a cough comes on sud-
> denly while your child is eating or playing with a
> small object, it is possible he has breathed some-
> thing into his upper airway.
>
> —THOMAS DALY, M.D.,
>   ST. JOSEPH'S CHILDREN'S HOSPITAL,
>   NEW JERSEY

If you do suspect that your child is choking, the ACEP
recommends that you first determine whether the child can
breathe, speak, or cough. If he can, don't do anything right
away, as coughing might dislodge the object. If your child is
not coughing, doctors recommend performing the appropriate Heimlich maneuver.

According to the Heimlich Institute, the instructions are
as follows:

1. From behind, wrap your arms around the victim's
   waist.
2. Make a fist and place the thumb side of your fist
   against the victim's upper abdomen, between the rib
   cage and the navel.

(continued)

3. Grasp your fist with your other hand, and press it into the abdomen with a quick upward thrust.

Repeat the procedure until the child expels the object, and stop if the victim becomes unconscious. For an infant, the instructions are similar, but the thrusts are given very gently, with the child sitting on your lap facing away from you. Instead of your fists, you use your thumb and forefinger.

Doctors recommend that every parent take a class in infant/child first aid and CPR, in case of emergencies.

Common causes of cough include asthma and allergies, and chest congestion or post-nasal drip from a respiratory infection. (See "Asthma," "Allergies," "Congestion," and "Stuffy Nose.") Cough might also be a sign that your child is choking on a foreign object.

If your younger child was playing with a small object and begins suddenly coughing, wheezing, or otherwise having trouble breathing, he might have swallowed or aspirated it. Seek medical attention right away.

—MURIEL WOLF, M.D.,
CHILDREN'S NATIONAL MEDICAL CENTER,
WASHINGTON, D.C.

Next, judge the severity of the cough, so you know if your child needs medical attention right away. If your child is showing signs of respiratory distress, such as gasping, extremely rapid breathing, chest heaving in, or nostrils flaring, call the doctor.

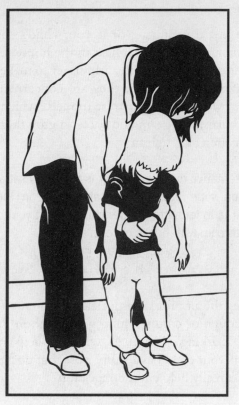

How to do the Heimlich Maneuver.

COMFORT CARE

As long as your child isn't having a respiratory emergency, simply look for the underlying cause of the cough. Then you can treat that or contact your doctor for assistance. Meanwhile, keep your child's throat nice and moist so she'll feel more comfortable.

Vaporizers

If you live in a dry climate, or if your child's cough comes during winter, when artificial heat in the house dries out the air, many doctors recommend a vaporizer to make your child more comfortable. However, they are concerned about the safety issues with the warm-mist models, which can cause accidental burns, and germ and bacteria growth in cool-mist models that aren't kept clean.

> One alternative to the vaporizer is to simply set a pan of water on your radiator or heat source on the floor. Another is to let a hot shower run and put your child in the bathroom with books or toys.
>
> —Carl Johnson, M.D., Ed.M.,
> Children's Hospital, Columbus, Ohio

Keeping the air moist is especially important if your child has a dry cough or croup, a lung inflammation that causes a distinctive "barking" cough. It will also help loosen nasal secretions if your child has a stuffy nose, but doctors contend that it won't really help chest congestion.

> Be careful about vaporizer overuse. Put the vaporizer on top of a piece of plastic to keep the moisture from getting into the carpet and causing bacteria to grow.
>
> —Helen Sinh-Dang, M.D.,
> Boys Town National Research Hospital,
> Omaha, Nebraska

Run the vaporizer all day in the room where the child sleeps, to keep moisture in the air; putting the vaporizer on only at night isn't adequate. Doctors recommend using distilled water and urge parents *not* to add medications of any type to the water. Both things could irritate your child's lungs.

Use vinegar and water to wash out cold-mist models every couple of days to fight bacteria that might be accumulated there.

—MURIEL WOLF, M.D.,
CHILDREN'S NATIONAL MEDICAL CENTER,
WASHINGTON, D.C.

If you are able to completely secure the vaporizer and keep it out of your child's reach, you might be able to get away with a warm-mist model, which is less likely to let germs and bacteria grow. However, if there is any chance that your child will come in contact with the vaporizer (and there's probably more chance than you think), go with a cool-mist model. Make sure vaporizers of any type are kept clean, so they don't serve as breeding grounds for irritants that might make your child's cough worse.

Liquids and Lollipops

Children with coughs and colds often have low-grade fevers (see "Fever"), may breathe slightly faster than usual, and may have decreased appetites. These things all mean they will become more dehydrated and therefore will need more fluids than usual. Many doctors say that whatever your child wants to drink is fine and will help keep him hydrated. Most people tend to prefer clear liquids when they are ill, and some drinks might seem less appealing. But the consensus is that if your child will drink it, it's fine.

There are many cultural beliefs about the nature, consistency, and temperature of fluids. In essence, these factors don't seem to make much difference.

—THOMAS DALY, M.D.,
ST. JOSEPH'S CHILDREN'S HOSPITAL,
NEW JERSEY

Don't give your infant an excessive amount of plain water, which has no salt or sugar content and might disrupt her electrolyte balance. Instead, give an electrolyte-replacement solution. If your baby is formula-fed and doesn't want to take her formula, you might try making it up as normal and then diluting it with electrolyte solution. However, don't dilute the formula with plain water.

—JOHN C. CARL, M.D.,
RAINBOW BABIES AND CHILDREN'S HOSPITAL,
CLEVELAND, OHIO

Most children older than six months don't want to drink the electrolyte-replacement solutions on the market, and doctors say they aren't necessary unless other factors are present, such as diarrhea (see "Diarrhea") or vomiting (see "Nausea and Stomachache").

White grape juice (because it doesn't stain if spilled) and electrolyte-replacement solutions are both good to give to prevent dehydration. You can dilute the electrolyte solution with juice to make it more palatable, but too much juice can cause diarrhea.

—MURIEL WOLF, M.D.,
CHILDREN'S NATIONAL MEDICAL CENTER,
WASHINGTON, D.C.

Doctors say that warm drinks, such as caffeine-free herbal tea (the kind that comes packaged in the grocery store, not loose in health food stores) or even warm water, can be soothing if your child likes them. It's easy enough to tell if your child is well hydrated; he'll likely be urinating every four to eight hours. If you suspect dehydration, contact your doctor.

Avoid citrus juices if your child has a sore throat.

—CHRISTOPHER WHITE, M.D.,
MEDICAL COLLEGE OF GEORGIA

There is no need to avoid milk. Contrary to popular belief, it does not thicken the nasal secretions. It only makes them appear white so that you can see them more easily.

—PHILIP FLOYD, M.D.,
MIAMI CHILDREN'S HOSPITAL

Your child's body has its own mechanisms for keeping the throat moist, and cough drops or hard candies can encourage these in older children. They will make your child swallow more frequently and breathe through her mouth, both of which work to keep the throat moist.

Be careful with cough drops or hard candies. Children can choke on them. Instead, you might try a lollipop, which is less dangerous and can make them just as comfortable.

—ELIZABETH PERKETT, M.D.,
CARRIE TINGLEY HOSPITAL,
ALBUQUERQUE, NEW MEXICO

Doctors seem to report no difference in effectiveness between medicated cough drops and simple hard candy, so use whatever your child prefers. Just make sure your child is old enough, and the cough is mild enough, that she won't choke.

Hard candies can be soothing, but kids under four or five can choke on them. These kids are better off having Popsicles, which have the same effect but also help get fluids into them.

—MURIEL WOLF, M.D.,
CHILDREN'S NATIONAL MEDICAL CENTER,
WASHINGTON, D.C.

If you give cough drops, make sure your child brushes
his teeth, as they usually contain a lot of sugar.
—CHRISTOPHER WHITE, M.D.,
MEDICAL COLLEGE OF GEORGIA

SYRUP SOLUTIONS

We've all seen the television commercial where the cough of
the adorable, stuffy-nosed child wakes the concerned mom,
who promptly goes into the room with bottle and teaspoon
and makes it all better so the family can sleep. However, doctors tend to report that unless Mom is carrying a bottle of
prescription cough medicine, the scenario is unlikely.

Still, the commercials and the plethora of available cold
preparations might tempt you to use over-the-counter medications if your child is coughing. Doctors' opinions seem to range
from fairly strict warnings against these products to comments
that they won't do much good but also won't harm if used as
directed. Doctors agree that you should never use over-the-
counter cough medications if your child is under a year old,
and that you should always follow dosing guidelines precisely.

Instead of medications, try warm lemonade, apple juice
or herbal tea [packaged, not loose] to soothe the cough.
Avoid antihistamines and decongestants if your child is
coughing. They only dry the lung tissue more. Also avoid
substances containing alcohol and aspirin.
—PHILIP FLOYD, M.D.,
MIAMI CHILDREN'S HOSPITAL

Over-the-counter cough remedies tend to come in three
basic classes: cough suppressants, expectorants, and combination medicines.

Expectorants, to be used in cases of "dry" cough, are designed to loosen phlegm so that it can be more easily coughed up and out of the airways. The common active ingredient in expectorants is guaifenesin. They do nothing directly to stop the cough, but are supposed to make the cough more "productive," so that the airways can be cleared and the child won't need to keep coughing. Doctors report that these are not very effective in children, so most physicians recommend against them.

> Give your child water to drink to help loosen the phlegm. It will work just as well as an over-the-counter expectorant, and it's cheaper.
> —HELEN SINH-DANG,
>   BOYS TOWN NATIONAL RESEARCH HOSPITAL,
>   OMAHA, NEBRASKA

How do you tell the difference between a dry and a wet cough in your child? A dry cough will probably sound more like he's trying to clear his throat, while a wet cough will sound like a rattle in the chest, and the child will often be coughing up phlegm.

Cough suppressants, as the name implies, work to keep the child from coughing. Doctors who recommend these tend to favor them mostly for nighttime use, and only if the child is having trouble sleeping because of the cough. The ingredient to look for in a good suppressant is dextromethorphan, found in brands such as Robitussin Pediatric Cough Suppressant and Benylin Pediatric Cough Suppressant, which is the only nonprescription ingredient doctors say is effective against cough. However, it works only in mild cases.

Don't use dextromethorphan if your child has asthma.
In a child with asthma, failure to cough could block the
airways.
>   —MURIEL WOLF, M.D.,
>   CHILDREN'S NATIONAL MEDICAL CENTER,
>   WASHINGTON, D.C.

Combination cough and cold medicines might contain
both an expectorant and a suppressant, plus decongestants,
fever reducers, and other medications. Doctors almost unani-
mously recommend against these, because the combinations
often have medications in subtherapeutic doses that won't help
but may still have side effects. You might give your child medications he doesn't need, or cause an overdose if you're using
one of these combinations along with other medications.

The labeling on cough and cold preparations can be confusing, and it's difficult for a parent to really tell whether
something contains an expectorant, a suppressant, or
both. Talk to your doctor or pharmacist to find out.
>   —CARL JOHNSON, M.D., ED.M.,
>   CHILDREN'S HOSPITAL, COLUMBUS, OHIO

It certainly doesn't make sense to use an expectorant and
a suppressant at the same time, as these are designed to work
in opposite ways. The expectorant can't encourage a productive cough if the suppressant is trying to stop the child from
coughing, and vice versa. Many doctors prefer that parents
use separate medicines for cough, congestion, and especially
fever. This way you know exactly what you are giving and
exactly how much, so you have less chance of overdosing or
giving unnecessary medications. You're unlikely to need a
prescription for an antibiotic to fight cough, since it won't
work against the viral infection your child likely has.

Doctors also remind parents that many over-the-counter medications, including those recommended as effective, have side effects that might interfere with appetite and sleep patterns. Don't use any preparation for more than two or three days without talking to your doctor.

OTHER THINGS YOU CAN DO

Aside from keeping your child hydrated or trying out an over-the-counter preparation, there is little you can do to treat your child's cough; it will go away when the underlying cause does.

> Propping your child's head up to keep secretions from pooling and triggering the cough can help. It's also good to stay with your child and read, chat, or do whatever you know makes her feel better.
>
> —CARL JOHNSON, M.D., ED.M.,
> CHILDREN'S HOSPITAL, COLUMBUS, OHIO

You can also help by removing irritants from the environment. These might include dust, smoke (even if you smoke only outside the house, you carry the residue in on your clothes), chemicals, perfumes, and strong soaps. Allergies could be the main cause of your child's cough, but even if they aren't, having these things in the air will make the cough worse.

> Gargling with warm salt water can be effective to soothe the throat. Put a pinch of salt in an eight-ounce glass of warm water, and try not to let your child swallow much of it. Corn syrup can also help for kids under four. Give one half to one teaspoon to swallow to coat and soothe the throat.
>
> —PHILIP FLOYD, M.D.,
> MIAMI CHILDREN'S HOSPITAL

If your child has been coughing a lot, her throat is also likely to be sore. Give her food and drink that will be soothing, and avoid those that might irritate.

Cough can also have an effect on appetite, especially in infants who might have a more difficult time eating.

If a cough is disrupting your infant's feeding schedule, you might want to divide the bottle and offer it over several small feedings, or offer the breast more frequently for a shorter period of time.

—CARL JOHNSON, M.D., ED.M.,
CHILDREN'S HOSPITAL, COLUMBUS, OHIO

In general, try to be soothing, comforting, and calm. Aggressive measures will just frustrate you both.

If you have a small baby who is coughing, don't pat her back. This is uncomfortable for infants. Instead, sit still with the baby on your lap, rub her forehead, and try to calm her down. The less you move her around, the more comfortable she'll be.

—HELEN SINH-DANG,
BOYS TOWN NATIONAL RESEARCH HOSPITAL,
OMAHA, NEBRASKA

WHEN TO CALL THE DOCTOR

If your child is coughing and seems to be having trouble breathing, it's a medical emergency and you need to find help right away. Call your doctor's urgent-care line, go directly to the emergency room or urgent-care clinic, or call 911. Your child might not be able to tell you something is wrong, but the signs are clear: breathing much faster than normal, wheezing or making an audible noise while breathing, and flaring nostrils. If the problem is severe enough, your child might even vomit or appear bluish in color. You also need immediate medical attention if your child has breathed an object into the lungs.

Even if the cough isn't interfering with your child's breathing, you might still need to call the doctor. A cough associated with a fever over 104 degrees Fahrenheit, or a fever that lasts more than three days, might be a sign of pneumonia. A cough that is high-pitched or sounds like barking might be a sign of croup. And a cough that goes on for more than ten to fourteen days could mean asthma, allergies, or a sinus infection.

The airways are lined with cilia—fibers that propel excess mucus out to the surface. When you have an upper respiratory infection, patches of these are torn away and the body has to cough to clear the mucus. It takes the body about three weeks to repair the respiratory system, which is why coughs tend to hang on after other symptoms have gone. But if the cough persists beyond that, there's the chance of another infection.

—JOHN CARL, M.D.,
RAINBOW BABIES AND CHILDREN'S HOSPITAL,
CLEVELAND, OHIO

Also call the doctor if the cough is painful, if your child is coughing up blood or excessive amounts of phlegm, or if the cough makes your child vomit. Even a relatively minor cough needs medical attention if it is so persistent that it impairs your child's normal activities, such as playing and sleeping.

Cuts and Scrapes

When I was about ten years old, I was hunting for polly-wogs in the park near our house, stepped on a piece of broken glass, and cut my foot. I limped the two blocks home, and my mom drove me to the hospital to get stitched up. The trail of blood on the sidewalk was famous in the neighborhood for weeks, and I lived to hunt pollywogs another day.

That was just one of the many instances when my mother was confronted with a bleeding child she had to bandage or drive to the hospital, which is to say that cuts and scrapes are part of childhood.

FIRST RESPONSE

TRIAGE

The first thing to do, as you are calming and comforting your child, is to assess the seriousness of the injury. Several factors will help you determine whether to go straight to the emergency room, call the doctor, or treat the cut or scrape yourself.

> The first thing to remember is not to panic, so you don't panic your child. If you can see a "pumping" blood vessel, put pressure on the wound and go to the emergency room.
>
> —MARK DIDEA, M.D.,
> ARNOLD PALMER HOSPITAL FOR CHILDREN
> AND WOMEN, ORLANDO, FLORIDA

If the wound is bleeding, place a clean rag or washcloth over it and apply firm, direct pressure for at least five minutes. Meanwhile, ask your child how the injury occurred. If the injury is from an animal or human bite, your child will need medical attention, because bites become infected easily and the wounds are often deeper than they look. Also call your doctor about any cut or scrape that happens around something dirty—such as trash or farm equipment—or if your child can't tell you how the injury occurred.

> Don't use the amount of blood to gauge the seriousness of a cut. Some parts of the body [such as the scalp] bleed quite a lot even with a small cut, and even a teaspoon of blood looks like a massive amount. The bigger concern is whether you can control the bleeding.
>
> —DAVID ROY KRONING, M.D., F.A.A.P.,
> ST. JOSEPH'S CHILDREN'S HOSPITAL,
> NEW JERSEY

Now check the wound to see if the bleeding has stopped. If it's still bleeding after ten minutes, call your doctor or urgent-care clinic, or go to the emergency room. If the wound has stopped bleeding, look at its size and shape.

A Stitch in Time

A cut is traumatic for most children, but the idea of going to the hospital for stitches is even worse. It's no picnic for parents, either, but don't delay if you have reason to believe your child's cut might require suturing. Doctors recommend that cuts be stitched within eight to twelve hours of injury: The skin will heal better, and there will be less risk of infection.

Whether it is best for a plastic surgeon or an emergency room doctor to stitch up your child's cut depends on both the comfort level and experience of the ER doctor, and the type of cut your child has, says W. Scott Colliton, M.D., of Children's Mercy Hospital in Kansas City, Missouri. "If, for instance, the ear, eyelid, nose, or lip is cut, most often the plastic surgeon is called in," he explains. "A simple cheek or forehead laceration would be considered reasonable for the ER doctor to do." Colliton also says that Dermabond, a "medical super glue," is sometimes used on small facial cuts. This lets your child avoid stitches altogether.

Don't give your small child anything to eat or drink on the way to the emergency room, in case she needs to be sedated.

—THERESA ANAYA, M.D.,
CARRIE TINGLEY HOSPITAL,
ALBUQUERQUE, NEW MEXICO

One way to make the experience easier for you both is to take your child to a hospital accustomed to dealing with children. The staff will be well versed in techniques for calming your child and explaining procedures that might seem frightening.

> Stay as calm as possible, because your attitude will be conveyed to your child. There's always room to hold your child's hand and speak calmly to him.
> —DAVID ROY KRONING, M.D., F.A.A.P.,
> ST. JOSEPH'S CHILDREN'S HOSPITAL,
> NEW JERSEY

No matter where you're going, bring along your child's favorite comfort toy, as well as other means of distraction. Be comforting but truthful, and don't tell your child it isn't going to hurt. A better approach is to explain why the stitches are necessary, that your child's pain will be worse without them, and that the doctor will use anesthetics to make sure it hurts as little as possible.

> If your child is very upset at the idea of having stitches, you can give him Benadryl to calm him down. Remember that you might be in the emergency room for a while, so bring favorite things for your child to do while he waits.
> —MARK DIDEA, M.D.,
> ARNOLD PALMER HOSPITAL FOR CHILDREN AND
> WOMEN, ORLANDO, FLORIDA

Doctors say it's worthwhile to ask the staff about topical painkillers to numb the hurt area before any shots are given. Some hospitals might also use staples, which some doctors say are easier and faster to apply and remove than traditional sutures, meaning a shorter procedure to endure.

(continued)

Stay with your child if you can handle it. But if you can't stay calm and collected, don't be there.

—TERRY ADIRIM, M.D.,
CHILDREN'S NATIONAL MEDICAL CENTER,
WASHINGTON, D.C.

If your child's cut is small and is in an area that doesn't get lots of movement, you might be lucky enough to qualify for Dermabond, a type of superglue for the skin. It requires no needles, no anesthetic, and no suture removal. If you do go home with stitches or staples, be sure to follow your doctor's instructions and care for them properly.

Stitches shouldn't be covered with bandages, but if your child picks at them, try covering the area with clothing.

—DEISE GRANADO-VILLAR, M.D., F.A.A.P.,
MIAMI CHILDREN'S HOSPITAL

Don't let your child pick at the stitches, and keep them dry. If the sutures get wet, they can actually absorb dirty water and pull it underneath the skin, which may cause an infection. If this happens, or if a stitch comes loose, call your doctor. Physicians say that some scarring is inevitable, so try not to stretch the wound, and go in to get the sutures out as soon as the doctor permits, to help keep the scar to a minimum. Delaying even a day can mean more scarring.

If the wound is more than an inch long, more than an eighth of an inch deep, or if the edges are jagged or gaping, the wound probably needs to be evaluated by a doctor. The location of the wound is also important. Wounds on the face, especially near the border of the lip, scar easily and require medical attention. Wounds on the joints should be treated by

a doctor, as well, because improper healing here can sometimes impair movement.

COMFORT CARE

If your child's wound isn't serious enough to merit a trip to
the doctor, your job as a parent is to "make it all better" yourself. Get the wound clean, apply a bandage if necessary, and
administer a healthy dose of TLC.

CLEANING

Doctors say that the longer you wait to clean a cut, the more
difficult it will be, so early cleansing of the wound is important.

> Cool compresses can help numb the cut or scrape
> before you clean it out. Products like Solarcaine or Ora-
> jel can also help, but shouldn't be used on abrasions
> larger than a softball, as this can cause too much lido-
> caine to be absorbed through the skin.
>
> —Mark DiDea, M.D.,
>   Arnold Palmer Hospital
>   for Children and Women,
>   Orlando, Florida

Good old-fashioned soap and water is all you will need
for this task. Don't reach for the isopropyl alcohol or hydrogen peroxide, as your parents might have. Doctors say that
these sting (remember?) and can even cause some tissue damage, making healing more difficult. Avoid harsh soaps or
detergents for the same reason.

If the cut or scrape has any foreign material—such as
gravel, splinters, broken glass, or dirt—embedded in it, and
you can't remove it with plain water and perhaps a little soap,

take your child to the doctor. Don't try to scrub the wound clean or remove the objects with your fingers or tweezers. You might end up making things worse.

> To clean a wound, hold the area under the tap (or shower, for larger areas), running with lukewarm water. Irrigating the wound this way is sufficient, and the fact that you are not actually touching the wound may make your child more comfortable with the process and more cooperative. Rubbing or scrubbing can make the wound worse.
>
> —THERESA ANAYA, M.D.,
> CARRIE TINGLEY HOSPITAL,
> ALBUQUERQUE, NEW MEXICO

BANDAGING

Most parents automatically bring out the bandages for cuts and scrapes. But doctors say this isn't necessary unless the cut or scrape in question is likely to get dirt in it or encounter friction. If it isn't, you can leave minor cuts and scrapes uncovered. However, a bandage is often the only way to keep a child's cut clean. It can also be used to keep an oozing cut from soiling clothing.

> You can't deprive a kid of an Elmo Band-Aid, but germs like to grow in a warm, dark environment, and that's what a bandage provides. So too much covering is not good.
>
> —CYNTHIA FERRELL, M.D.,
> DOERNBECHER CHILDREN'S HOSPITAL,
> PORTLAND, OREGON

If you're going to bandage a cut, do so only for the first few days. After the wound has begun to heal, leave it open to the air so it can begin to dry out and scab over.

Some doctors recommend applying an antibiotic ointment to minor cuts as an added protection against infection. Choose the right size bandage for the job, so the cut is covered by the gauze and not the adhesive tape, which might stick to the wound and cause more damage during dressing changes.

Make sure to choose a dressing that won't stick to the wound. Buy nonadherent gauze, then put an ointment over the cut to help keep the skin from sticking.
—DAVID ROY KRONING, M.D., F.A.A.P.,
ST. JOSEPH'S CHILDREN'S HOSPITAL, NEW JERSEY

To remove self-adhesive bandages, lift the edge and apply some baby oil. Wait a minute, and the bandage will come right off.
—DEISE GRANADO-VILLAR, M.D., F.A.A.P.,
MIAMI CHILDREN'S HOSPITAL

Be sure to remove any bandages and clean the wound on a daily basis. This way you can see what the wound is doing, make sure it is healing well, and look for signs of infection.

To steri-strip a small cut, attach both strips to one side of the cut, then pull them across the cut so that the skin on one side of the cut overlaps the skin on the other. The skin needs to be dry for this to work. If you're taping a cut, run the tape perpendicular to the way the large muscle—for instance, the ones that run the length of your arm or leg—runs. It will stay on better.
—MARK DiDEA, M.D.,
ARNOLD PALMER HOSPITAL
FOR CHILDREN AND WOMEN,
ORLANDO, FLORIDA

Some small cuts will do well bandaged with steri-strips, small adhesive strips that hold the edges of the cut together. But doctors advise that these strips work well only with small cuts that have clean edges and are in locations that don't scar easily and aren't subject to much movement. If you have any doubt as to whether the steri-strips are adequate for your child's cut, call your doctor.

Make It Better

You can try a variety of things to ease the pain of a cut or scrape. One of the simplest and most readily available for young children, is to have your child "blow away the pain." This is a simple distraction technique that encourages deep, regular breathing, focuses attention away from the cut, and might help calm your child down while you bring other measures into play. Have your child pretend to blow out candles, blow up a balloon, or blow to spin a pretend pinwheel.

Ice is another fast and simple pain reliever, but doctors warn that it shouldn't be put directly on the skin. Besides being uncomfortable for your child, it can damage tissue and actually make things worse. Instead, insulate the ice in a washcloth, towel, or clean rag. Better yet, use a cold compress or ice water.

There are also many over-the-counter gels and sprays that contain lidocaine and other pain relievers. Some doctors recommend them in small doses but warn against overuse. Because the lidocaine is absorbed through the skin, a child can easily get an overdose if it is used on a large area or in large amounts; this can lead to seizures and other serious consequences.

There isn't much in the literature regarding dosage ranges for lidocaine, especially for children. I recommend a three- to four-hour use with application with something like a cotton swab. Parents shouldn't use lidocaine-containing products on an as-needed basis. This seems to be where I have seen younger children get into trouble.

> —DONALD J. FILLIPPS, M.D.,
> SHANDS CHILDREN'S HOSPITAL AT THE
> UNIVERSITY OF FLORIDA

Don't apply aloe or vitamin E to an open wound. You don't want oils in the wound that will block the cleaning. Wait until a scab starts to form before using them.

> —DEISE GRANADO-VILLAR,
> MIAMI CHILDREN'S HOSPITAL

You can also give an oral over-the-counter pain reliever such as acetaminophen (Tylenol) or ibuprofen (Advil). Both are widely considered safe and effective, but doctors are divided over which to choose. Some consider ibuprofen a marginally better pain reliever, while others say acetaminophen is less likely to upset the stomach or cause a mild increase in bleeding. Others have no preference. If in doubt, call your pediatrician and ask what she prefers.

As It Heals

If scabbed knees are a rite of childhood, so is picking off the scabs. Your job as a parent is to keep the picking to a minimum, as it can lead to infection and scarring.

Keep your child's fingernails cut short and his hands clean, and do your best to keep him distracted so he doesn't pick at wounds, scabs, or stitches. Apply vitamin E as the wound heals to help decrease itching.

> —CYNTHIA FERRELL, M.D.,
> DOERNBECHER CHILDREN'S HOSPITAL,
> PORTLAND, OREGON

Keep the wound soft and moist once the scab has started to form. You can use antibiotic ointments or other creams to help, but don't use lidocaine or hydrocortisone creams, which can damage tissue and actually impede healing.

Soak abrasions in warm water and gently pat them dry once they've been healing three to four days. This will soften the scab and help the healing process. Be careful with newly healed tissue, as it is easily damaged. Protect it from the sun and from harsh chemicals.
—MARK DiDEA, M.D.,
ARNOLD PALMER HOSPITAL
FOR CHILDREN AND WOMEN,
ORLANDO, FLORIDA

Moisturizing and vitamin creams will do their job only if used continually until after the scab is completely gone. If you let the wound dry out, it will crack and itch again, and your efforts will have been in vain. To help prevent scarring, keep the healing area out of the sun as much as possible.

WHEN TO CALL THE DOCTOR

If your child's wound is on the face or joints, or is large, ragged, gaping, or bleeding profusely, you'll want to call the doctor. Two other factors also merit immediate medical attention, or at least a call to the doctor: signs of infection, or the possibility that your child needs a tetanus shot.

Doctors say that signs of infection generally will appear three to five days after the initial injury. Extreme redness, heat, pus, continued pain, or red lines radiating from the wound might mean your child has an infection around the injured area. Fever and irritability could be signs that the infection is systemic, meaning it has spread to the rest of your child's body.

If your child has even a mildly serious cut, be sure his vaccinations are up to date. Children under five might need a tetanus shot and a tuberculosis booster, and kids over age ten who haven't had boosters might also need them. The shot needs to be given within twenty-four to forty-eight hours of the injury. If you are in doubt, doctors advise that your child should have the shot.

Diaper Rash

If diaper changes are no fun for new parents, they're nothing compared to how unpleasant diaper rash can be for babies. The skin is designed to be dry, and when we diaper our babies, we're basically marinating their sensitive skin in acidic urine and stool, which causes irritation and "diaper dermatitis," the most basic kind of diaper rash. The diaper itself holds in moisture and creates a nice, warm, wet, dark place where bacteria, yeast, and fungus can grow and cause secondary infections that create a more serious rash.

On top of this, chemicals in the diaper wipes we use to clean baby's bottom, or in the diaper itself, can cause further irritation. No one does this on purpose, of course. But it's an unfortunate fact that if you have a baby, she will at some point have a diaper rash.

FIRST RESPONSE

PAIN IN THE BUTT

Diaper rash can make a baby extremely uncomfortable and fussy, so your first priority is to try to soothe the irritated skin. Try a warm sitz bath—a bath taken sitting in a basin, so that the water covers only the hips and buttocks—or a soak in a warm tub, which is comforting and increases circulation to the area to promote healing.

> Applying a liquid antacid that coats the skin can help soothe the pain of diaper rash. You can also try putting half a cup of vinegar in a partially full bathtub, or about a tablespoon in a baby tub. This helps soothe the skin and get its pH back to normal.
> —Mary K. Rogers, M.D., F.A.A.P.,
> Carolinas Medical Center

Meanwhile, you can give the appropriate dose of acetaminophen, or whichever over-the-counter pain reliever you use with your baby. This usually takes half an hour to kick in, so it should start working just after the bath is over.

> If your child's skin is very irritated, use a plant sprayer and water to spritz the baby clean, or dunk her in a tub. This way you don't even have to touch the skin.
> —Nancy VanderSluis, M.D.,
> Boys Town National Research Hospital,
> Omaha, Nebraska

After the bath, let your baby's bottom air-dry well, and apply a coat of soothing petroleum jelly or diaper cream before diapering. Some doctors say that hydrocortisone cream can also be soothing, but you shouldn't use it for more than a day or two without talking with your doctor, because of danger that the skin will atrophy, or start to shrink.

Once you've taken some steps to soothe the rash—and hopefully to calm your baby and make him feel a bit more comfortable—you can use what many doctors call "preventive diapering" to help heal this rash and prevent future problems.

COMFORT CARE

Your efforts to clear up existing diaper rash, and to prevent your child from having it again in the future, should center around keeping your child's bottom as clean and dry as possible. This means frequent diaper changes, properly cleaning and drying the diaper area with each change, and applying "barrier" creams as needed to keep urine and stool away from the skin.

PREVENTIVE DIAPERING

The most important and helpful thing you can do to prevent diaper rash, according to doctors, is to change your child's diaper frequently. During the day, your baby will need changing as often as every two hours, or about eight times a day—and maybe even more frequently if you are using cloth diapers. If your baby's diaper is soiled, change it immediately; avoid the temptation to wait to see if the baby is going to poop or pee again right away. Make sure that anyone caring for your child does the same.

The Diaper Decision
The type of diaper you choose can also make a difference, though not as much as how frequently you change it. When

you aren't able to change your child's diaper immediately—
for instance, if you're out with the baby, or if the baby is
asleep—doctors say that disposables are best at keeping moisture away from the skin. Keep in mind that even disposables
won't keep stool away from the skin, and that soiled diapers
always need to be changed right away.

> The superabsorbent disposable diapers on the market
> are really helpful in keeping moisture away from the
> baby's skin. If your baby is really prone to diaper rash,
> cloth diapers won't keep the moisture away from the
> skin nearly as well as the new disposables.
>
> —LISA GELLES, M.D.,
> THE CHILDREN'S MEDICAL CENTER OF DAYTON

If you choose disposables, doctors recommend that you
pay attention to the brand you buy: different diapers contain
different chemicals. If you use disposable diapers and your
baby is having trouble with diaper rash, sometimes another
brand can make a difference. On the other hand, if you've
just changed brands and your child starts getting diaper rash,
you might want to change back. A chemical in the diaper
itself could be causing irritation.

> If you're having trouble with diaper rash and are laun-
> dering cloth diapers at home, boil them. There are
> many types of bacteria that can live through washing
> and drying.
>
> —NANCY VANDERSLUIS, M.D.,
> BOYS TOWN NATIONAL RESEARCH HOSPITAL,
> OMAHA, NEBRASKA

If you choose cloth diapers and wash them at home
rather than using a diaper service, be certain to wash them in

hot water and rinse well to remove all traces of detergent. Detergent residue can irritate your baby's skin and contribute to diaper rash.

> Rinsing cloth diapers with vinegar and water will acidify the diaper and help neutralize the ammonia in the urine. When you do this, don't follow with a plain-water rinse. If you're washing diapers at home, it's also better to use simple detergents, rather than heavy-duty ones.
>
> —MARY K. ROGERS, M.D., F.A.A.P.,
> CAROLINAS MEDICAL CENTER

To Wipe or Not to Wipe

No matter what type of diaper you use, you'll be faced with cleaning up your baby's diaper area with every wet or dirty change. This, doctors say, is a balancing act.

On one hand, you need to be thorough enough to make sure your baby's skin is completely clean; any urine or stool that is left on the skin can irritate. On the other, you need to be gentle enough not to irritate the skin with friction.

> Don't scrub your baby's skin to clean it. Stay away from diaper wipes that contain alcohol, and if your child is prone to diaper rash, don't use soaps that have perfume. Lots of baby soaps contain perfume, so concentrate on the "sensitive skin" lines to be safe.
>
> —LISA GELLES, M.D.,
> THE CHILDREN'S MEDICAL CENTER OF DAYTON

Most doctors say that diaper wipes are fine if your child doesn't have a rash, but are best avoided if she does. Instead, use a washcloth or soft paper towel and some warm water to clean your baby's diaper area.

If your child has or is prone to rash, avoid diaper wipes. These contain either glycerine or lanolin, which are moisturizers that trap moisture in the skin. If there is a rash, the skin needs to be kept dry.

—NANCY VANDERSLUIS, M.D.,
BOYS TOWN NATIONAL RESEARCH HOSPITAL,
OMAHA, NEBRASKA

Even if your child doesn't have a rash, cutting back on the use of wipes is a good idea. Some parents tend to think they need to use two or three wipes to clean up after every wet diaper, but the chemicals and the scrubbing can irritate the skin. Use a damp cloth instead, and save the wipes for the big jobs.

Definitely Dry

To prevent diaper rash, your child's skin has to be dry as well as clean. Air is the best way to dry. "The main problem in the diaper area is that the skin is occluded [smothered]," says Lisa Gelles, M.D., of the Children's Medical Center in Dayton, Ohio. "If you can air the diaper area, that's a great remedy for almost any problem down there." Indeed, many doctors seem to think that in an ideal world, little bottoms could just go diaperless. This, of course, isn't practical much of the time.

Let your child air-dry after a bath or change where you've used a wet wipe. Be sure not to put the diaper back on until the skin feels dry to the touch. Moisture left on the skin could lead to yeast infection.

—SHARON D. VERMONT, M.D.,
ST. LOUIS CHILDREN'S HOSPITAL

It would also be great if you could leave the diaper on loosely to allow extra air to get at the skin, but loose diapers leak. The best you can do is just air your baby's bottom whenever practical. Put down an old blanket or towel to catch the spills, and leave the diaper off for a while.

> Moisture on your baby's skin tends to stay there, especially if it gets trapped in crevices. You can air-dry, blow-dry (with a hair dryer on the "cool" setting), or use Kleenex or toilet tissue to blot dry.
>
> —NANCY VANDERSLUIS, M.D.,
>   BOYS TOWN NATIONAL RESEARCH HOSPITAL,
>   OMAHA, NEBRASKA

> If you're using cloth diapers, don't double up on plastic pants. This keeps the area so airtight that diaper rash is more likely.
>
> —MARY K. ROGERS, M.D., F.A.A.P.,
>   CAROLINAS MEDICAL CENTER

Take a Powder?

There was a time when baby powder was found on every changing table, and it always went on with a fresh diaper. However, research during the past several years has shown that the talc found in many types of powder is a carcinogen and can cause pneumonia if it gets into your baby's lungs.

> I've heard of some parents using baking soda or boric acid directly on the skin. Don't use these, as they can be toxic.
>
> —LISA GELLES, M.D.,
>   THE CHILDREN'S MEDICAL CENTER OF DAYTON

There are new cornstarch powders that don't contain talc but could still be breathed into baby's lungs. Some doctors also express concern that cornstarch could contribute to the growth of yeast in the diaper area. Other doctors say that this hasn't been proven but that cornstarch is still worth avoiding if your baby is prone to yeast infections.

> Caldescene, which has an antifungal ingredient, is a good powder if there's a problem with fungal infection.
>
> —MARY K. ROGERS, M.D., F.A.A.P.,
> CAROLINAS MEDICAL CENTER

Powders decrease moisture and help prevent friction, so some doctors still recommend them, especially in the crease areas right after a bath. These doctors caution parents not to "go crazy with it" or to shake the powder into the air. The best way to keep the powder out of baby's lungs is to shake a small amount into your hand, then apply it to the diaper area. Also be careful to keep the powder container out of your baby's reach, so that he doesn't grab it and shake powder loose.

Build a Barrier

Not every child needs diaper cream every day, but if your child has a rash or is on the way to getting one, you need to create a barrier between that nice dry skin and the inevitable flooding of the diaper.

> If your child's bottom looks at all red, put a barrier cream on to prevent diaper rash. However, your child doesn't need this after every single change.
>
> —SHARON D. VERMONT, M.D.,
> ST. LOUIS CHILDREN'S HOSPITAL

Doctors say that the main element of most diaper creams is either zinc oxide, a drying agent, or petroleum jelly, which repels moisture. Both of these things, in their generic form, work just fine. However, with so many good over-the-counter diaper-rash creams available, doctors encourage parents to try a different cream if the one they're using isn't working well.

> Plain petroleum jelly provides a good barrier and is probably the best thing to help prevent and treat diaper rash. Zinc-oxide ointments are also good, but they are more tenacious. They are harder to wipe on and off of irritated skin. Vitamin A and D ointment has vitamins mixed with petrolatum, which can help heal the skin.
>
> —MARY K. ROGERS, M.D., F.A.A.P.,
> CAROLINAS MEDICAL CENTER

No matter what type of cream you're using, you want to put it on at the first signs of rash, and enough to truly protect your child's skin from urine and stool. If you don't use enough, doctors say, you might as well not use any at all.

> Plain zinc oxide is a good diaper cream and less expensive than name brands. Put enough on to create a "clown face" effect, so that your child's bottom looks as white as a clown's face. Remember that some of the cream will be soaked into the diaper.
>
> —DALE ANN CODDINGTON, M.D.,
> CHILDREN'S NATIONAL MEDICAL CENTER,
> WASHINGTON, D.C.

YUCKY YEAST

Doctors say that the longer a diaper rash lasts, the greater the chances are that the area will become infected with fungus as well. Yeast infections—also known as candida—in the diaper area won't respond to the treatment you would give a normal diaper rash, so it's important that you learn to tell the difference.

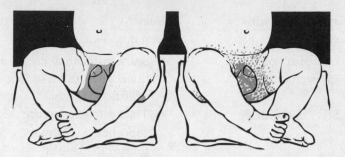

Diaper dermatitis vs. yeast infection.

Rash-Busting Recipes

At Carolinas Medical Center, they have a couple of "special recipes" that doctors favor for treating particularly stubborn cases of diaper rash. "Sometimes kids have a little bit of fungal infection along with some contact irritation," says Mary K. Rogers, M.D., F.A.A.P. "These two recipes are especially good if your child has a combination of factors going on."

ROSEN 123 OINTMENT

> 10cc Burrow's solution
> 20g Aquaphore
> Enough zinc oxide to make a total of 60g

GREER'S GOO

> Equal parts: Zinc oxide
> One-percent hydrocortisone cream
> Mycostatin (antifungal) cream

Though all of the ingredients are available over the counter, Rogers recommends that you have a pharmacist mix them to guarantee accurate measurements. A small drugstore is more likely to do it than the big chains, Rogers says. You can also take the recipe to your pediatrician and ask him or her to write a prescription for you.

Diaper Dermatitis	Yeast
• Mild red in color	• Bright "beefy" red
• Uniform color and appearance	• Scaly, with small circles at the edge; looks like "lots of little red dots"
• Stays in the diaper area	• Tracks up toward the abdomen and down toward the thighs
• Can begin anywhere in the diaper area	• Usually starts in the creases of the skin

Be especially careful to look for signs of yeast infection if your baby has oral thrush (a yeast infection in the mouth), or if she is on antibiotics, which can increase chances of yeast infection.

When applying prescription cream to diaper rash, put it on first, then cover it with a barrier cream to hold in the medication and keep out urine and stool. The prescription medication won't act as a barrier.

—DALE ANN CODDINGTON, M.D.,
CHILDREN'S NATIONAL MEDICAL CENTER,
WASHINGTON, D.C.

If a routine diaper rash lasts longer than two days without beginning to improve, that's another sign that yeast may be involved. Doctors say that over-the-counter antifungal creams are safe and effective. However, if the antifungal cream you've tried doesn't help within two or three more days, see your pediatrician, who can prescribe something stronger.

WHEN TO CALL THE DOCTOR

Most diaper rash can be treated easily and successfully at home. However, if your home treatment isn't working, if your child's rash seems to be getting worse or is spreading to other parts of the body, or if your baby is in severe pain, it's a good idea to call the doctor.

Skin in the diaper area that is broken, bleeding, or scabbed increases the chances of a secondary infection. The doctor can evaluate the seriousness of the rash and prescribe antibiotics if needed to prevent or fight off infection. If your child's skin has yellow, crusty blisters, she might have impetigo—a bacterial infection of the skin—and will need to see the doctor in case a prescription antibiotic is needed.

Even if your child's diaper rash seems to be fairly "normal," call the doctor if you can't seem to clear it up in a few days, or if the rash never completely goes away.

Diarrhea

As common as it is unpleasant, diarrhea eventually afflicts all of us—and our kids. Whether it's from a viral infection being passed around the family or the schoolyard, an antibiotic prescription to treat an ear infection, or something that didn't agree with your child's digestive system, there's not much to do besides let it run its course.

Doctors define diarrhea as an increase in the frequency, fluidity, or volume of stool. If your child generally has three bowel movements a day and now he's having seven, he probably has diarrhea. Doctors say that true diarrhea is watery, and that the severity of a case is usually judged by the frequency of the stools. If your child is having more than eight bowel movements in eight hours, it's considered severe.

FIRST RESPONSE

INCREASE FLUID INTAKE

Diarrhea robs the body of essential fluids and can lead to life-threatening dehydration if it goes unchecked. So the first thing to do if your child has diarrhea is to start increasing his fluid intake. Offer small amounts of fluids as frequently as possible, and watch for signs that your child is becoming dehydrated—such as infrequent urination, or crying without tears.

Hydration, Hydration, Hydration

The main danger associated with diarrhea is dehydration. In fact, there are still some places in the world where dehydration caused by diarrhea kills a significant number of children each year. Doctors take it seriously, especially in very young children. Dehydration is more difficult to prevent if your child has high fever or vomiting as part of the same illness, so doctors warn parents to be especially watchful in these cases.

Child's weight	Fluid needed every 24 hours
11 lbs.	17 oz.
22 lbs.	33 oz.
33 lbs.	42 oz.
44 lbs.	50 oz.
55 lbs.	53 oz.
66 lbs.	56 oz.
77 lbs.	60 oz.
88 lbs.	63 oz.

(continued)

If your child is losing fluid through diarrhea, you'll need to give enough fluid to replace what's lost, plus keep up with the regular daily amount she needs.

You can tell how much fluid a baby is losing by weighing the dirty diaper and subtracting the weight of a clean diaper.

—ERENA TRESKOVA, M.D.,
ST. JOSEPH'S CHILDREN'S HOSPITAL,
NEW JERSEY

Doctors say you cannot rely on a child's thirst to keep him hydrated if he is losing lots of fluid through diarrhea. Instead, it's better to have some idea of how much fluid your child needs, and make sure he gets it.

Give over-the-counter oral rehydration solutions slowly and frequently, about one teaspoon every five minutes. With babies, you can use a medicine dropper or syringe to make it more convenient.

—ROY E. BROWN, M.D.,
COLUMBIA PRESBYTERIAN MEDICAL CENTER

You shouldn't try to give all this fluid at once, especially if your child has an upset stomach. Divide it into manageable amounts and give small portions frequently.

In Babies

If you are breast-feeding, continue to offer the breast if your baby has diarrhea; increase the frequency of feedings to help keep your child hydrated. If the diarrhea is severe, offer oral rehydration solution between feedings as well, and seek medical attention.

Don't give boiled skim milk, which is an old home remedy for diarrhea. It has too much salt in it and so can upset your child's electrolyte balance. For the same reason, don't give too much plain water, which

can take salt from the body and upset the balance
the other way.

—MATILDA GARCIA, M.D.,
ST. JOSEPH'S HOSPITAL AND
MEDICAL CENTER, PHOENIX

If your baby is formula-fed, doctors advise against diluting formula with water, and differ on whether or not it should
be diluted with oral rehydration solution. For mild diarrhea,
many recommend full-strength formula and oral rehydration
solution as a supplement. Others suggest preparing the formula as normal with water, then diluting it with oral rehydration solution. Still others say that you should discontinue
formula and give one or two bottles with just electrolyte solution; next, give one or two bottles of half-strength formula,
then work your way back to full-strength formula.

In Older Kids

If your child is older and has mild diarrhea, many doctors say
you can give her whatever fluids she wants to drink. Clear liquids are often best tolerated, especially if your child's stomach is upset, but stay away from drinks that are too sugary, as
they can irritate the digestive tract and can actually make the
diarrhea worse.

Kids like sports drinks better than children's oral
rehydration solutions, but sports drinks have more
sugar. If your child won't drink the oral rehydration
solution, you can dilute a sports drink with water, or
give alternate sips of sports drink and water to cut
down on the amount of sugar.

—JILL REEL, M.D.,
BOYS TOWN NATIONAL RESEARCH HOSPITAL,
OMAHA, NEBRASKA

You don't need to start giving oral rehydration solution
at the first loose stool, but do take precautions: Give extra

(continued)

fluids to prevent dehydration, and dilute sugary drinks such as apple juice with water. If the diarrhea becomes more serious, you might need to encourage your child to drink oral rehydration solution, or even try some of the oral rehydration ice pops on the market.

> You can add about a quarter to a half teaspoon of Kool-Aid powder per cup to oral rehydration solutions to make them more palatable.
>
> —GLENN C. ROSENQUIST, M.D.,
> CHILDREN'S NATIONAL MEDICAL CENTER,
> WASHINGTON, D.C.

Remember that the oral rehydration solution will not cure the diarrhea; it will only help prevent dehydration.

Signs of Dehydration

The clearest sign that your child is dehydrated is lack of urine output. If your baby needs fewer diaper changes than usual, or your older child is going to the bathroom less frequently to urinate, pay close attention. If your child hasn't urinated in six to eight hours, she is dehydrated, and you should call the doctor.

Other signs of dehydration include dry mouth and crying without making tears. Don't wait for these symptoms to show up before you increase your child's fluid intake. However, if they are present, get your doctor's advice right away. It's possible that your child is dehydrated to the point that extra fluids alone will not be enough.

CATCH THE CAUSE

Another important consideration is determining what might have caused the diarrhea. The most common cause by far, according to doctors, is rotavirus, a viral infection that almost everyone has had at least once by age three. This "bug" may go around your child's school, or even around your family, and is highly contagious. For this reason, common disease-prevention measures like handwashing are essential if someone in your family is ill.

It's also possible, though less likely, that the diarrhea is from a bacterial infection such as salmonella. This is the bacteria found in undercooked meat and eggs, and it is more serious than a case of rotavirus. So stop and consider what your child has been eating, or whether you recently traveled out of the country to someplace where salmonella and intestinal parasites are more common. If you suspect your child has a salmonella infection or a parasite, seek medical attention.

Another fairly common cause of diarrhea in young children, according to doctors, is too much juice in the diet. If your child frequently has bouts of diarrhea, take a look at his amount of juice intake and try cutting back. A less common dietary cause is dairy intolerance, which usually appears very early in life, and so is less likely to show for the first time in an older child. Diarrhea is also sometimes a side effect of antibiotics prescribed to children for things like ear infections.

Antibiotic-Associated Diarrhea

Many of the common antibiotics used to fight childhood infections can also cause bouts of diarrhea. These cases are usually mild and last just a day or two.

Unless the diarrhea is severe, doctors recommend that you continue to give the medication as prescribed. Just take some common comfort measures, such as cutting back on fruit juices and offering a gentle diet. Be especially careful about diaper rash in babies and skin irritation in older children.

If the diarrhea is severe, stop giving the medication but call your doctor right away. Keep track of antibiotics that have caused diarrhea in your child, so that you can request alternatives next time your child is ill and needs antibiotic treatment.

While you're gathering information, make a note of how many times a day your child is having diarrhea, so that you can share this information with your doctor if necessary.

COMFORT CARE

If the diarrhea doesn't appear to be from a serious infection, and your child is taking in plenty of fluids and staying hydrated, the best thing to do is "wait out" the illness as comfortably as possible. This means a diet that is easy on the digestive system, dealing with cramps, and preventing skin irritation.

DIET TIPS

Assuming your child's stomach can handle food, and that she is willing to eat, doctors recommend basically sticking with her normal diet, along with a couple of minor changes that should make things easier on your child.

> Milk isn't particularly good for kids with diarrhea, but if it's the only thing your child will drink, go ahead and give it to her. Having some milk to drink is better than getting dehydrated.
>
> —JILL REEL, M.D.,
> BOYS TOWN NATIONAL RESEARCH HOSPITAL,
> OMAHA, NEBRASKA

Avoid giving large amounts of fruits or fruit juices and foods that are high in sugar and fat. Gravies and sauces are a big culprit here; they tend to make the diarrhea worse. Also avoid spicy and fried foods, which will likely irritate an already irritated digestive system. Large, heavy meals, which are hard to digest and harder on the system, are probably not a good idea, either, and likely won't be appealing to your child.

There are now infant formulas with some rice cereal added. These are excellent if your child has diarrhea.

—Matilda Garcia, M.D.,
   St. Joseph's Hospital and Medical Center,
   Phoenix

The BRATY diet is idea for children with diarrhea who will eat. This means bananas, rice, applesauce, toast, and yogurt. The yogurt helps replace the normal bacteria that is washed out of the digestive system by the diarrhea. It's the natural way to get it back into the system.

—Roy E. Brown, M.D.,
   Columbia Presbyterian Medical Center

For a baby on solids, many doctors recommend rice cereal, which sometimes helps slow down the diarrhea. In a child over a year, in addition to BRATY foods, you can encourage breads, cereals, mashed potatoes, and other starchy foods such as crackers. When she feels a little better, you can give some lean chicken breast or other lean cuts of meat.

The most dangerous myth about diarrhea is the one that says, "Put the gut to rest." It used to be thought that you shouldn't feed a child with diarrhea for a period of time. However, doing this can disrupt the child's electrolyte balance.

—Matilda Garcia, M.D.,
   St. Joseph's Hospital and Medical Center,
   Phoenix

Doctors stress that while a child with diarrhea might not be up to eating his normal diet, it's important for him to eat something. If a child is fed only clear liquids for two or three days, he may have green, watery stools. These are called "starvation stools" and mean the child is not getting enough nutrition. If your child is vomiting as well and is unable to keep food down, or completely refuses to eat, contact your doctor.

THE BOTTOM LINE

Along with the dangers of dehydration and the discomfort to the stomach, diarrhea can also cause abdominal cramps and make your child's skin irritated and sore. So while you're keeping your child hydrated and providing a gentle diet, you'll also want to keep her skin clean and protected, and to try and ease the pain of cramps.

> A warm water bottle against the abdomen will help ease cramps. But test the temperature against your cheek before giving it to your child, to prevent burns and scalds.
> —ERENA TRESKOVA, M.D.,
> ST. JOSEPH'S CHILDREN'S HOSPITAL, NEW JERSEY

To prevent skin irritation, make sure that your child's skin is completely clean and dry after each bowel movement. A sitz bath, with water in a basin to just cover the hips and buttocks, or even a quick bath in a regular tub, is good for this, and some kids find it soothing. You can also gently clean the area with a washcloth and warm water. Let the skin air-dry, or pat dry carefully and thoroughly with a towel.

> Using an over-the-counter diaper cream, even in older kids, can help soothe and protect the skin from irritation.
> —SHARON D. VERMONT, M.D.,
> ST. LOUIS CHILDREN'S HOSPITAL

Once the skin is clean, coat and protect it with a barrier cream such as petroleum jelly, to keep the stool away from the skin during your child's next bowel movement.

If your baby has diarrhea, change diapers as often as possible to avoid soreness and diaper rash. Wipes can make the irritation from the stool worse, so don't use them. Use warm water to clean the skin very gently instead.

> —JANET KLEPEK, D.O.,
> RONALD McDONALD CHILDREN'S HOSPITAL
> OF LOYOLA

None of the herbal antidiarrheal medications on the market has been studied in children. Don't use them without consulting your doctor.

> —ERENA TRESKOVA, M.D.,
> ST. JOSEPH'S CHILDREN'S HOSPITAL, NEW JERSEY

Acetaminophen (Tylenol) is the only over-the-counter medication doctors say is okay to give your child for diarrhea. Medications that slow the passage of diarrhea won't actually cure it or prevent fluid loss; the fluid will escape another way. Stopping the diarrhea will only mask this symptom of illness and might actually prolong it by keeping the digestive system from clearing itself.

WHEN TO CALL THE DOCTOR

As long as you're keeping your child well hydrated and comfortable, many cases of diarrhea can be safely left to run their course. Unfortunately, this can take as long as two weeks, which can seem like much longer when you have a sick child on your hands.

If you have an infant less than three months old, or an immunocompromised child, call your doctor at the first signs of diarrhea because of the greater risk of complications. Otherwise, just watch for signs that something more serious is going on.

If there is blood or mucus in your child's stool, or if she's in extreme pain, a more serious illness is likely at work, and you should call the doctor. High fever and persistent vomiting are signs that something is wrong, and they pose an increased risk that your child will become dehydrated—another reason to seek medical attention. Also call if your child becomes lethargic or is just acting very ill.

If no other complications seem to be present, give the doctor a call if your child's diarrhea lasts more than a week, or if he begins losing weight because of it: This could mean the illness won't go away without medical treatment.

Earache

The most common cause of ear pain in children is otitis media, an infection of the middle ear. Tiny tubes running from the ear into the throat, called the eustachian tubes, become blocked, and the fluid they would normally allow to drain from the ear builds up and becomes infected. The fluid pushes against the eardrum, causing pain. Most doctors treat otitis media with a course of oral antibiotics (since many strains of bacteria are becoming resistant to antibiotics, some doctors are electing not to prescribe them in every case). Doctors overwhelmingly agree that parents should follow their pediatrician's advice where antibiotic treatment is concerned.

Another frequent cause of ear pain is an infection of the skin in the ear canal. Known as otitis externa, or swimmer's ear, it is prevalent in older children who spend a great deal of time in the water. These infections are treated with antibiotic eardrops.

Signs of ear pain can include irritability, fever, sleeplessness and lack of appetite, or pain when the outer ear is moved. Most doctors agree that pulling or tugging at the ear is not cause enough to suspect infection; however, if your child is experiencing other symptoms as well, it might be a sign worth noting.

Ear pain can strike at any time of day, but children with ear trouble tend to be more symptomatic between eight P.M. and three A.M., probably because lying down increases pressure in the ears and intensifies the pain.

FIRST RESPONSE

OVER-THE-COUNTER PAIN RELIEVERS

Antibiotics, the prescribed treatment for most causes of ear pain, need at least forty-eight hours to take effect. Until you can get your child to the doctor to begin treatment, over-the-counter pain relievers are a good way to ease your child's discomfort.

Ibuprofen and Acetaminophen

Ibuprofen (sold under the brand names Motrin and Advil) and acetaminophen (Tylenol) are the two major classes of nonprescription pain reliever available for children. Ibuprofen is the most recommended medication, and the best at true pain relief in the presence of acute inflammation.

Ibuprofen, in the experience of many pediatricians, is the longer-lasting of the two. It can be given every six hours and lasts about six hours. Acetaminophen, on the other hand, can be given every four hours but generally lasts only three. Ibuprofen is probably the one to try first—especially at night, to allow your child to get a good night's rest. If you give acet-aminophen, you may find yourself getting up in the middle of the night to give another dose.

However, if your child has a sensitive stomach, an allergy to aspirin (which would also mean she's allergic to ibupro-fen), or has been having stomach upset connected with a cold or flu, acetaminophen is probably a better choice, since it does not have the potential side effect of stomach irrita-tion. Doctors also recommend staying away from ibuprofen if your child is going to have surgery in the near future since ibuprofen thins the blood and could cause excessive bleeding.

> To get the best effect from ibuprofen or acetamino-phen, call your doctor with a good estimate of your child's weight, so you can learn the maximum dose you can give your child. You can also "layer" the two prod-ucts for a day or two if neither seems to be doing the job alone. Start with ibuprofen, then four hours later, give a dose of acetaminophen. Alternating the two products every four hours is safe because acetamino-phen is cleared from the body by the liver, while ibupro-fen is cleared by the kidneys.
>
> —JANET M. BELTON, M.D.,
> ARNOLD PALMER HOSPITAL FOR
> CHILDREN AND WOMEN,
> ORLANDO, FLORIDA

Be sure not to exceed the maximum recommended dose for either product, and do not give more than is recommended in any twenty-four-hour period. An overdose of acetamino-phen can cause life-threatening liver damage.

Analgesic Eardrops

Eardrops, such as Auralgan or Americaine—available by pre-scription—might also be worth asking for if your child is complaining of ear pain. Some parents swear by them. They can be effective against both middle-ear infections and swimmer's ear, and usually provide relief within two minutes. Doctors caution against using the drops if the child's eardrum is perforated, since they can cause severe pain if they get behind the eardrum. However, ear pain is rarely a symptom of a perforated eardrum, because perforation relieves both the pressure and pain inside the ear.

Proper technique in preparing and placing the drops can increase their effectiveness.

First warm the drops as close as possible to body temperature by holding the bottle or dropper in your hand, or under warm water from the tap, for a few minutes. Not warming the drops could increase your child's discomfort, increasing pain or even causing dizziness.
—ROBERT O. RUDER, M.D.,
CEDARS-SINAI MEDICAL CENTER, LOS ANGELES

Have your child lie down on her side. The couch in front of the TV is an ideal place, since placing the drops during a commercial and keeping your child still until the next commercial will allow plenty of time for the drops to begin working. It takes only a second for the drops to coat the ear canal.
—JANET M. BELTON, M.D.,
ARNOLD PALMER HOSPITAL FOR
CHILDREN AND WOMEN,
ORLANDO, FLORIDA

Place the drops so that they run along the side of the ear canal, rather than trying to drop them straight into the center. This allows the ear canal to fill from the bottom up, and prevents trapped air from blocking the canal and stopping the medication from reaching the eardrum.

—MICHAEL MACKNIN, M.D.,
CLEVELAND CLINIC CHILDREN'S HOSPITAL
FOR REHABILITATION

Analgesic eardrops, available by prescription, can be used until antibiotics have cleared the infection. Doctors caution that if you have some left over from a prior infection, you should not use them in lieu of making an appointment with your pediatrician.

Not Recommended

Aspirin: Pediatricians generally warn parents against giving aspirin to children—especially children who might have a viral infection—because of the danger of Reye's syndrome, a potentially life-threatening illness that often requires hospitalization.

Decongestants/Antihistamines: Doctors also advise against giving over-the-counter cold medications to children under age six. "They don't open up stopped-up ears, nor do they prevent colds from turning into ear infections," says A. Larry Simmons, M.D., of Arkansas Children's Hospital, adding that the antihistamines often found in these medications tend to thicken nasal secretions and may even make an infection more likely. In older children, decongestants might help treat the stuffy nose that often comes in conjunction with an ear infection (see "Congestion"). However, they will not help clear up middle-ear fluid.

Over-the-counter pain medications can take up to thirty minutes to relieve pain. In the meantime, several home remedies can soothe and comfort your child.

Warm Compresses

Local heat in the form of a heating pad can offer great relief of pain and have a wonderful soothing effect in the presence of an earache, especially in the wee hours when nothing else is available. It can also be used with ibuprofen, Tylenol with codeine, and other prescribed remedies.

—JAMES LABAGNARA, JR., M.D., P.A., F.A.C.S.,
ST. JOSEPH'S CHILDREN'S HOSPITAL, NEW JERSEY

Apply warm compresses for ten to fifteen minutes at a time, taking care not to let the heating pad or compress get too hot—especially with infants.

—SCOTT R. SHAFFER, M.D., F.A.C.S.,
THE CHILDREN'S REGIONAL HOSPITAL AT COOPER,
CAMDEN, NEW JERSEY

Warm Oil

Another way to warm up a child's ear is with mineral oil. Place the container of oil into a glass of hot tap water for several minutes to bring it to a warm but not hot temperature, and place several drops in the painful ear. An additional benefit of using warm oil is that it may work to soften excess ear wax, making it easier to remove when the pediatrician needs to look into the ear.

—DAVID E. KARAS, M.D.,
YALE–NEW HAVEN CHILDREN'S HOSPITAL

If your child won't stay still to let the warm oil do its work, try putting cotton into the ear to keep the oil in place. Be careful not to force the cotton into the ear canal.

—RAVINDRA RAO, M.D.,
LOMA LINDA UNIVERSITY CHILDREN'S HOSPITAL

Elevating the Head

Raising your child's head, either by having him sit upright or by placing extra pillows under his head and shoulders, can sometimes reduce the intensity of the pain in much the same way that elevating an injured extremity relieves pressure and pain.

—A. LARRY SIMMONS, M.D.,
ARKANSAS CHILDREN'S HOSPITAL

The most effective way to keep an infant's head elevated is to hold the baby in an upright position, perhaps against your shoulder, while rocking her. Your touch will be an added comfort. It may also help to have the child avoid lying on the affected ear.

The Balloon Trick

If your child is old enough to follow directions, holding her nose while she tries to blow up a balloon might help relieve ear pain caused by otitis media or eustachian-tube dysfunction (where the tubes are blocked but no infection is present) by equalizing the pressure in the ear temporarily. It might even allow some of the fluid trapped in the ear canal to drain. This works most effectively if the child does it a few times in succession every five or ten minutes.

—ROBERT O. RUDER, M.D.,
CEDARS-SINAI MEDICAL CENTER,
LOS ANGELES

Removal of Ear Wax

Parents often take great pains to keep their child's ears clean and to remove any excess wax. But they are probably doing more harm than good. Ear wax serves a protective function and becomes a problem only when someone is trying to look in the ear. Clearing the wax from the ear is unnecessary unless it is impairing your doctor's vision or your child's hearing. Wax and dirt visible on the outside of the ear can be cleaned with soap and warm water.

> Do not use Q-tips to clean your child's ears. They counteract the normal flow of wax out of the ear, pushing the wax deeper into the ear canal. Excessive use of Q-tips can actually cause infection of the skin in the ear canal.
>
> —JAMES S. REILLY, M.D.,
>   ALFRED I. DUPONT HOSPITAL FOR CHILDREN,
>   WILMINGTON, DELAWARE

If your pediatrician does need to see inside your child's ear, she may clear the ear herself, or she may want you to tackle the job. In that case, there are several things you can try.

> Put drops of a warm hydrogen peroxide and water solution (in equal parts), or warm mineral oil, into the ear to loosen the wax, then rinse the ear with warm water.
>
> —ROBERT ZAVOSKI, M.D., M.P.H., CONNECTICUT
>   CHILDREN'S MEDICAL CENTER

> Try a commercially available ear wax–removal kit, which contains eardrops that can be used to soften the hardened wax. This can later be followed by gentle irrigation with a bulb syringe and a half warm water–half vinegar mixture.
>
> —ANNA MESSNER, M.D.,
>   LUCILE PACKARD CHILDREN'S HOSPITAL
>   AT STANFORD

DEALING WITH THE SIDE EFFECTS
OF ANTIBIOTICS

Many antibiotics cause side effects, the most common being
diarrhea and upset stomach. Keep a record of each type of
antibiotic your child has taken, noting any such reactions.
That way, if your doctor prescribes an antibiotic that doesn't
agree with your child, you can ask her to prescribe something else. With the wide range of antibiotics in use, there is
almost always an alternative available.

PREVENTING SWIMMER'S EAR

Otitis externa, also known as swimmer's ear, is not as likely a
cause of ear pain as otitis media. But if your child spends a lot
of time in the water and has had frequent otitis externa infections, there are preventive measures.

Mix a solution of half rubbing alcohol and half white vinegar (acetic acid). Use five drops in the affected ear after
swimming. The vinegar solution changes the pH balance
of the ear, which helps prevent bacteria from growing.

—SCOTT R. SHAFFER, M.D., F.A.C.S.,
THE CHILDREN'S REGIONAL HOSPITAL AT COOPER,
CAMDEN, NEW JERSEY

A half-and-half mixture of hydrogen peroxide with vinegar will also work as a preventive measure.

—ROBERT ZAVOSKI, M.D., M.P.H.,
CONNECTICUT CHILDREN'S MEDICAL CENTER

Doctors say that parents should not try either mixture
unless they have a child who has been previously diagnosed
with swimmer's ear, since changing the pH balance of an
uninfected ear isn't recommended.

Use of Home Otoscopes

A number of otoscopes have been marketed to parents for at-home use. They are sold under the premise that parents can look into their child's ear and determine whether she has a buildup of fluid or an ear infection.

Doctors, however, consider them a waste of money, saying that a parent's inexperienced eye is unlikely to accurately detect an ear infection. "New residents in pediatrics and oto-laryngology will admit that they must examine hundreds of ears (and sometimes more) before they are sure of the subtle nuances in both normal and infected ears," says James LaBagnara, Jr., M.D., P.A., F.A.C.S., of St. Joseph's Children's Hospital in New Jersey. And even the average pediatrician is wrong 30 to 40 percent of the time in detecting ear fluid, according to Michael Macknin, M.D., of Cleveland Clinic Children's Hospital for Rehabilitation.

In addition, the generally poor quality of these scopes, which often sell for less than half the price of professional models used by pediatricians, makes them inadequate as a diagnostic tool.

WHEN TO CALL THE DOCTOR

Ear pain that lasts more than forty-eight hours after your child begins treatment for an ear infection merits a return to the doctor. Other signals that current treatment isn't working—or that an ear infection may have spread beyond the ear—include high, unresponsive fever, unusual headaches, sensitivity to light, refusal to eat or drink, seizure, inability to walk, crooked smile, or any asymmetry of the face. You should also consult your pediatrician if there is redness or swelling behind your child's ear, or if the ear seems to be sticking out from the head at an unusual angle.

But there could be a much more subtle sign that something is wrong. If your child is unusually irritable, lethargic, or "if they're really not themselves," David E. Karas, M.D., of Yale–New Haven Children's Hospital says, a return visit is in order. "When a parent says something is different this time, that's when I say I want to see them. And a significant proportion of the time, it's something real," says Karas.

ASSESSING DRAINAGE FROM THE EAR

Alarming as it may seem, blood or pus on your child's pillow or draining out of her ear may not necessarily warrant a return trip to the doctor. Such drainage occurs when a child's eardrum perforates, and doctors point out that this is a natural part of the healing process. If the discharge concerns you, or if your child exhibits other symptoms, you may want to call your doctor.

> Don't panic if your child's eardrum perforates. Even though it looks awful, because there may be lots of pus and blood draining out of the ear, it generally provides the child with a great deal of relief.
> —MICHAEL MACKNIN, M.D.,
> CLEVELAND CLINIC CHILDREN'S HOSPITAL
> FOR REHABILITATION

LINGERING FLUID IN THE EAR

Once a course of antibiotics has been completed, usually after a week to ten days, pediatricians generally follow up to make sure the infection is cleared. But the antibiotic only fights the infection; it doesn't work to clear the fluid. Even after the ear is no longer infected, it is common for some fluid to remain for as long as two to three months. This does not mean your child needs another course of antibiotics, unless the fluid becomes reinfected.

At your follow-up visit, ask your pediatrician if fluid is still present. Do not request another course of antibiotics unless there is still an infection.

—ANNA MESSNER, M.D.,
LUCILE PACKARD CHILDREN'S HOSPITAL
AT STANFORD

Be aware that the fluid will affect your child's hearing, and take extra care to make sure you have her attention when speaking to her. Inform your child's teacher so that she can be moved nearer the front of the classroom if necessary.

—MICHAEL MACKNIN, M.D.,
CLEVELAND CLINIC CHILDREN'S HOSPITAL
FOR REHABILITATION

It's rare for hearing loss due to ear fluid to be permanent. See your pediatrician if your child's hearing isn't back to normal a few months after the infection. Also consult the doctor if your child develops symptoms that seem to suggest reinfection.

Fever

When my daughter, Lauren, was around two years old, my husband and I had tickets to see a Frank Sinatra concert. We had imported my mom to baby-sit for the occasion, and when Lauren developed a slight fever, I was relieved that it was Mom who would be watching her for the evening. My relief turned to disappointment when Mom announced that under no circumstances would she watch a child with a fever. Around the same age, I had had a frightening febrile seizure and a trip to the hospital. My mother was taking no chances on going through that again.

Doctors, however, report that seizures are rare, and that fevers in and of themselves are nothing to be afraid of. They are merely one of the body's many mechanisms for dealing with illness.

Febrile Seizures

Febrile seizures are the most common seizures of childhood, but that doesn't make them any less frightening. And though this type of seizure generally isn't dangerous and produces no lasting effects, parents have no way of telling whether it is the result of fever or something else. For this reason, always notify your doctor if your child has had a seizure.

While the seizure is going on, make sure your child doesn't hurt himself. This means clearing away furniture or other objects on which he might hit his head, and helping him to lie down gently on his side. If your head remains clear enough, glance at your watch and try to time the seizure.

If you can and if it makes sense, loosen your child's clothing to make him more comfortable. Then call for emergency medical assistance.

If your child has a seizure, don't try to drive him to the hospital yourself, even if the seizure has passed. Call 911. Your child might have another seizure, which would be dangerous in the car. You could also endanger your family if you try to drive while you are upset.

—MATTHEW O. McKEEVER, M.D.,
CHILDREN'S NATIONAL MEDICAL CENTER,
WASHINGTON, D.C.

Don't put anything in your child's mouth, try to hold a wildly struggling child still, or panic and create a scene. Stay as calm as you are able, and be prepared to give as much information to the emergency personnel as you can about what your child was doing when the seizure began and how long it lasted.

Your child's doctor will be able to give you instructions regarding what to do if your child ever has another seizure.

FIRST RESPONSE

NUMBER, PLEASE?

You might have begun with the classic hand to the forehead, but you'll eventually have to resort to the thermometer to determine your child's temperature. How difficult that is depends on your child's temperament; how necessary, on your child's age.

If you have an infant—especially one under three months of age—doctors need the most accurate temperature possible. One of the most common causes of a fever is the body trying to fight off an infection of some sort. In infants, doctors might not have other signs of that infection and will have few ways to find out what it might be. Temperature is a crucial factor in deciding whether involved tests such as blood work or even a spinal tap might be needed. A rectal temperature is the only way to get a truly accurate reading in an infant. Ear thermometers, forehead strips, and other gadgets just won't do the trick.

> If you use an electronic thermometer of any kind (including digital), check it once in a while to make sure it is working properly. If the battery has run out, or it's broken, it might freeze at an inaccurate temperature. The only way to check some models is to take someone else's temperature with them and make sure you get a different reading.
>
> —ALBERT FINCH, M.D.,
> CHILDREN'S HOSPITAL OF THE KING'S DAUGHTERS,
> NORFOLK, VA

Taking a rectal temperature is fairly easy until your child reaches a year and a half. Luckily, getting an absolutely accurate reading is much less important by this time than during the infant years. When your child is too big for a rectal temperature but not yet able to sit still for an oral thermometer, doctors say it's fine to take an axillary temperature under the arm, or to try one of the newer ear thermometers or fever strips that go on the forehead. These readings might not be as accurate as one from a more traditional thermometer, but they will work for your needs and your doctor's.

> If you're using an ear thermometer and the reading doesn't seem to match the way your child is feeling to the touch, take his temperature using another method. If your child has an ear infection, the eardrum will be hot, and this will yield an inaccurate ear thermometer reading.
>
> —HELEN SINH-DANG, M.D.,
> BOYS TOWN NATIONAL RESEARCH HOSPITAL,
> OMAHA, NEBRASKA

Once your child reaches the age of four or five and is old enough to follow your instructions, she's ready for an oral thermometer.

In general, doctors seem to prefer mercury or digital thermometers. The ones who recommend digital over mercury do so because mercury thermometers are more difficult to read. All types of thermometers need to be cleaned before and after each use, and the mercury types need to be shaken down below 96 degrees Fahrenheit before use.

> Read the manufacturer's recommendations to decide how long to leave the thermometer in place. Different thermometers require different amounts of time, and this is the only way to tell for certain about your particular thermometer.
>
> —MICHAEL LAMACCHIA, M.D.,
> ST. JOSEPH'S CHILDREN'S HOSPITAL, NEW JERSEY

The only other trick to taking a temperature is to keep your child still and quiet for the two or three minutes. Unless your child is under three months old—in which case you should call your doctor if there is any fever at all—your final task is not to get too excited about the thermometer reading. Doctors agree that what your child is doing is more important than what the thermometer is doing.

> As a parent, you should have a sense of how your child generally acts when he's ill. If that's the way he's acting, even with a fever of 104 degrees Fahrenheit, there's probably no reason to worry.
> —RUBY ROY, M.D.,
> RONALD MCDONALD CHILDREN'S HOSPITAL
> OF LOYOLA

A child with a high fever who is playing and otherwise acting normally is of less concern than a child with a low-grade fever who appears very ill. "Brain damage from fever can't happen until about 108 degrees Fahrenheit, and illnesses don't create temperatures that high," says Roxanne Kane, M.D., of Children's Hospital of Wisconsin. "About the only things that could drive fever that high would be leaving a child in a very hot car, or a reaction to medication." So unless your child has a fever around the 105 mark, you don't need to call your doctor unless she seems very ill. And in that case, you're concerned about the illness rather than the fever itself.

COMFORT CARE

If your child doesn't have symptoms that merit a call to the doctor, then the only reason to try to lower her fever is to make her more comfortable. Doctors say that because we live in a fast-fix society, a lot of parents think it's bad if they can't completely get rid of the fever. The thing to remember is that in lowering a fever, you're making the child more comfortable, but you're not treating the disease.

Doctors say most people won't be uncomfortable until their fever reaches around 103 degrees Fahrenheit.

COOL AND COMFY

A good place to start if you're trying to lower your child's temperature is to make her environment cooler and more comfortable. Make sure she's wearing loose and comfortable clothing, and put her in as little as she is contented wearing. Don't undress her so much that she's shivering; just enough that she isn't overheated. The only reason you're lowering the fever is to make her more comfortable, so there's not much point in making her uncomfortable in the process.

Many doctors still recommend sponge baths or tepid baths to lower fever, but caution against anything that cools the body too quickly. Doctors also warn against rubbing-alcohol baths, because of the added danger of poisoning from alcohol absorbed through the skin.

> The mistake most parents make when giving a tepid bath is that they don't leave the child in there long enough. He needs to stay in there twenty to thirty minutes to really lower his temperature.
>
> —KENNETH KATZ, M.D.,
> COLUMBIA PRESBYTERIAN MEDICAL CENTER

Anything that makes your child so cold he shivers is going to drive the fever even higher and end up making him more uncomfortable. So keep baths lukewarm, not cold. And if your child complains, give up what you're doing.

Wrap an ice bag or a bag of frozen vegetables in a towel and put it on the back of her neck. This is a much gentler way to lower the temperature.

—HELEN SINH-DANG, M.D.,
BOYS TOWN NATIONAL RESEARCH HOSPITAL,
OMAHA, NEBRASKA

If your child is old enough to understand, ask him what he wants to do. If a cool cloth on the forehead or a bath sounds good, go ahead. Otherwise, just do whatever seems to work for your child's comfort level.

HYDRATION

You can also help lower your child's temperature—and help prevent dehydration—by giving cool liquids to drink. When the body is feverish, it tends to lose more moisture than normal. And if your child is vomiting (see "Nausea and Stomachache") or has diarrhea (see "Diarrhea") along with the fever, he's even more likely to need extra fluids.

Your child is less likely to throw up if you give fluids that aren't too heavy. Clear liquids such as apple juice, water, or even Gatorade are usually best.

—ALBERT FINCH, M.D.,
CHILDREN'S HOSPITAL OF THE KING'S DAUGHTERS,
NORFOLK, VIRGINIA

If your child is eating without vomiting or having bouts of diarrhea, then doctors say he can have whatever fluids he normally drinks. This means that babies can have formula or breast milk as usual, and older children can have the beverages you routinely offer.

If your child doesn't want anything to drink, try offering her a Popsicle as a way to sneak in some extra fluids.
—Roxanne Kane, M.D.,
Children's Hospital of Wisconsin

If your child isn't able to keep down food and drink, or is refusing meals, doctors recommend giving an oral rehydration solution instead of other beverages. These will help your child replace needed salts and sugars in the body in a way that plain water cannot.

To make the oral rehydration solution more palatable, chill it thoroughly and give it in very small doses at a time. You can also mix it with flat soda to help mask the taste.
—Helen Sinh-Dang, M.D.,
Boys Town National Research Hospital,
Omaha, Nebraska

Whatever you're offering to drink, it's probably best to offer small amounts and frequently. Even if your child is thirsty, having too much to drink at once could upset her stomach. You'll get more fluids into her if you take it a little at a time.

OVER-THE-COUNTER MEDICATION

If other measures aren't helping and your child is still uncomfortable, doctors suggest giving the appropriate dose of an over-the-counter fever reducer. Most recommend either acetaminophen (children's Tylenol) or ibuprofen (children's Motrin or Advil). Both of these are generally considered safe and effective; both have their advantages and disadvantages.

Acetaminophen, which has been around longer and is more familiar to both doctors and parents, is the easier of the two on the stomach. However, its effects generally last just four hours. Ibuprofen, which is considered by some doctors to be stronger and a bit more effective, lasts up to six hours, but it is more likely to irritate the stomach.

Give whichever of these medications has worked best for and been tolerated best by your child. Whichever you give, read the label carefully, measure the dose accurately, and follow it up with plenty of water.

In cases where a child has pain, doctors often recommend that you alternate acetaminophen and ibuprofen, giving a dose of one, then a few hours later a dose of the other. However, it is risky to do this if your child has fever. Doctors report that many parents lose track of which medication they gave when, especially if they are worried and busy tending a sick child, and this can cause an accidental overdose. Damage from overdose is even more likely if the body is dehydrated from fever and the liver and kidneys are forced to process more concentrated doses of medication.

Doctors also urge parents to avoid giving aspirin to children, because of the danger of Reye's syndrome, a potentially fatal complication.

UPS AND DOWNS

Once they've discovered that their child has a fever, and they've taken measures to lower it, most parents want to check and recheck to see if the fever is going down. Doctors say that this doesn't need to be done as frequently as most parents believe. Unless you have a young infant with a high fever, in which case she should be under a doctor's care, you really don't need to check the temperature unless your child seems to be feeling uncomfortable.

In fact, doctors say that some parents overmedicate their child in their zeal to bring down the fever. They give medication and recheck the temperature after fifteen minutes, and if the fever hasn't come down, they decide to give more medication. This could lead to overdose. Doctors tend to agree that as long as your child seems to be doing fine, taking the temperature once in the morning and once at night is adequate. This will help you keep track of how many days your child has had fever, which is more important at this point than the fever's ups and downs.

> If you've put your child to bed and she's sleeping and seems to be doing all right, don't wake her up just to take her temperature or give her over-the-counter medication. Fever is the body's response to illness; don't expect it to go away with one dose of Tylenol.
> —SUSAN M. MONK, M.D.,
> THE CHILDREN'S MEDICAL CENTER OF DAYTON

Remember that a fever isn't determined by numbers alone. Normal temperature varies from person to person, and can even vary within an individual by as much as a degree throughout the day, so you probably don't need to concern yourself with minor variances if your child is otherwise fine. In the words of Albert Finch, M.D., of Children's Hospital of the King's Daughters, Norfolk, Virginia, "Most of these unpleasant kinds of symptoms have good purpose to them. Don't worry about the fever; wonder why the child has the fever."

WHEN TO CALL THE DOCTOR

Of course, there are times when a child with a fever needs medical attention. These usually have to do with the age of your child, the level or duration of the fever, or the symptoms that go along with it.

If you have an infant under a year, seek medical attention any time the baby has a fever, even a fairly mild one. Fevers are signs of illness, and almost any illness in a young baby is potentially serious.

If your child at any age has a fever of 104 degrees Fahrenheit or higher, give the doctor a call. The fever itself isn't dangerous, but one this high can be a sign of the type of infection or illness that requires medical treatment. The same is true if your child has a fever that won't go down despite the appropriate dose of over-the-counter medication, or if the fever doesn't improve within three days. These are signs of an illness that won't get better on its own.

Even if your child's temperature isn't very high, or she hasn't had the fever very long, call the doctor if she is acting markedly different than normal. Symptoms such as headache, stiff neck or reluctance to move her head, rash, cough, or sore throat often indicate an illness serious enough for medical attention—something beyond a routine cold or flu. Dehydration caused by fever also requires medical treatment. Also call if your child seems to have no symptoms, so that you can't tell what might be causing the fever, or if your child doesn't feel better even after the fever comes down. This means there's another cause of discomfort that your doctor should look into.

Headache

You might think of headaches as a grown-up problem, but there's every chance your child doesn't. Somewhere around 5 percent of kids get headaches, so the problem is fairly common, says Jerome Esser, M.D., of Children's Hospital of Wisconsin. Luckily, the vast majority of them aren't caused by anything serious.

In fact, the most common cause of headache in children is your run-of-the-mill viral illness. This is especially true in children under the age of five or six. Colds and the flu can make kids achy all over, and the headaches generally go away when the infection does.

Doctors tend to see even more headaches in older kids; these can be caused by tension or migraine as well as illness. Tension and migraine headaches tend to be recurrent. According to William McClintock, M.D., of Children's National

Medical Center, at least 10 percent of ten-year-olds get headaches once a month or so. Headaches can also be caused by sinus or dental pain, though this is rare. There are no actual nerves in the brain, so what we perceive as head pain always comes from another source.

How Bad Does It Hurt?

It can be difficult to get children to explain what type of headache pain they're having, or how badly it hurts. While older children can describe the pain they are having in detail, you might have to help younger kids along. You can try asking them to put their pain on a scale of one to ten, or use a scale of faces—from smiley face to crying face—to indicate the level of pain.

To gather information about your child's headaches, use the "W"s.

- Where on the head is the pain?
- When are the headaches occurring?
- What type of pain and symptoms does your child have?

—SIEGFRIED SCHMIDT, M.D., PH.D., F.A.F.P.,
UNIVERSITY OF FLORIDA COLLEGE OF MEDICINE

If your child isn't able to say more than that it hurts, try putting the following list in front of her:

- Pounding
- Sharp
- Cutting
- Burning
- Like a tight band around the head
- Squeezing
- Head feels like it's bursting
- Pulsating

(continued)

Be careful—especially with younger children—not to ask leading questions, because they are liable to just say yes to whatever you describe. Instead, tell them their headache might be completely different from any one of these, but that some kids have headaches that feel like the things on the list. Ask them if their pain matches any of the words.

You can illustrate different types of headache. I sometimes take my fist and hit my hand repeatedly to show a child what I mean by "pounding." Even older kids might not be able to describe their pain. You'll have to ask them questions like "Is it pounding? Is it sharp? Is it a constant pain?"

—FRED BOMBECK, M.D.,
COLUMBIA PRESBYTERIAN MEDICAL CENTER

However, it's just as important (and easier) for parents to note how much disability the headache caused. Could the child play or do any other activities? Could he read or watch TV, or did he have to lie down in a dark room? If your child is able to continue with what he was doing at the time the headache began, it isn't likely very intense.

If your child is under age six or seven, take everything he says about the severity of the headache or type of pain with a grain of salt. Kids this age aren't very good at describing pain. To help, you can ask questions such as "If you were playing when you got your headache, would you stop? If you were at school, would you have to come home?"

—WILLIAM MCCLINTOCK, M.D.,
CHILDREN'S NATIONAL MEDICAL CENTER,
WASHINGTON, D.C.

FIRST RESPONSE

KNOW YOUR CHILD'S HEADACHE TYPE

Because headaches are a symptom of some other problem in the body, the best way to treat them is to find out the cause. Treating or removing the underlying cause will often help the pain go away. Unless you know that your child is prone to headaches not associated with illness, the first thing you should do is look for symptoms of a cold or flu. Helping your child recover from the illness will generally stop the headaches.

> It is important to know where the headache is, where the head is hurting. Pain at the back of the head often means tension headaches. Pain at the sides is usually migraine. Pain at the front is often sinus.
>
> —JEROME ESSER, M.D.,
> CHILDREN'S HOSPITAL OF WISCONSIN

If your child isn't ill, the headache is probably from tension or migraine. Tension headaches come from muscular problems that are usually stress-related, just like in adults. Remove the stress and you'll improve the headache.

> Kids don't always complain about their headaches. If your child comes to you saying that he has a headache, ask if he has had one before, and get the details.
>
> —WILLIAM McCLINTOCK, M.D.,
> CHILDREN'S NATIONAL MEDICAL CENTER,
> WASHINGTON, D.C.

Migraine headaches are vascular, which means they come from a blood-flow problem, and can occur in children as young as two or three. They usually occur in response to triggers, such as types of foods or hormonal changes associated with the menstrual cycle. If the trigger can be avoided or minimized, the headache will improve.

COMFORT CARE

A simple headache usually requires simple treatment. Getting your child into a comfortable environment, offering a cold compress and a gentle massage, or giving a dose of over-the-counter pain reliever is often enough. However, if your child's headaches are recurrent, lifestyle changes might be in order.

HEADACHE FIRST AID

Changing the Environment

The first thing many doctors recommend is that you take a look at where your child was and what he was doing when the headache began. Running around in the hot sun or playing loud video games could have contributed, so you should move your child to a more comfortable environment. A cool, quiet room is probably a good place to start.

> The first thing to try if your child complains of a headache is to let him lie down in a dark room. Offer to put a cold compress on his head, and try to calm and soothe him.
>
> —WILLIAM MCCLINTOCK, M.D.,
> CHILDREN'S NATIONAL MEDICAL CENTER,
> WASHINGTON, D.C.

Keep in mind that other measures aren't likely to do much good if your child stays in the environment that caused the headache in the first place. Even if you give medication, it isn't likely to work if your child goes back out into the sun to play rather than resting.

Sleep is one of the best treatments for migraine. Sometimes just putting the child down to rest in a cool, dark
room, giving her an analgesic, and even giving her a dose
of Benadryl to help her sleep, will do the trick. Children
get some sleep and they wake up feeling better.

—FRED BOMBECK, M.D.,
COLUMBIA PRESBYTERIAN MEDICAL CENTER

Medication

If rest in a comfy place isn't working on its own, try the appropriate dose of over-the-counter children's pain reliever. Most
of these contain either acetaminophen, such as in Tylenol; or
ibuprofen, such as in Motrin or Advil. Doctors say that in general, both of these are safe and effective. Pressed to recommend
one over the other, many say that acetaminophen is good to
try first because it is less likely to cause upset stomach. However, many also say that ibuprofen is a bit stronger and lasts
longer, and is a good choice if it doesn't bother your child's
stomach. All doctors warn parents against giving products containing aspirin, because of the danger of Reye's syndrome, a
potentially fatal complication.

Don't give analgesics for a first headache that lasts
under an hour if you aren't sure what's causing it. It will
mask the symptom, and you won't be able to tell the
cause or whether the headache would have gone away
by itself. However, if you know your child gets recurrent
headaches, give medication right away. Analgesics are
much more likely to be effective if you give them immediately.

—POORVI PATEL, M.D.,
ST. JOSEPH'S CHILDREN'S HOSPITAL, NEW JERSEY

The idea when using medications is to treat as early as possible with a strong dose to knock the headache out. Dosing is

crucial. Never give more medication than is recommended for your child's age and weight, but it's also a bad idea to give less.

> Using both acetaminophen and ibuprofen can be very effective. You can alternate every few hours. This can be especially helpful if your child has vomiting with the headache (which children often do) and is vomiting up doses of medication. If you've just given a dose of ibuprofen, for instance, and your child vomited, you don't have to guess at the new dose. You can safely give a full dose of acetaminophen to replace what was lost. Just be careful not to overdose the child with either product.
>
> —FRED BOMBECK, M.D.,
> COLUMBIA PRESBYTERIAN MEDICAL CENTER

Many parents don't like to give too much medication, so they wait too long and then underdose. A couple of hours later, when the medication hasn't proved effective, they give a little bit more, and over the course of twenty-four hours they end up giving much more medication than if they'd given the correct dose in the first place.

> Over-the-counter medications can give rebound headaches if you overuse them. This can be an especial problem if the family doesn't make the needed lifestyle changes but instead relies on the medications. Don't use them for more than two days per week.
>
> —SIEGFRIED SCHMIDT, M.D., PH.D., F.A.F.P.,
> UNIVERSITY OF FLORIDA COLLEGE OF MEDICINE

Doctors also caution against using over-the-counter headache medications daily; this practice can cause rebound headaches, which occur when the child doesn't get the medication. If you find yourself giving your child an over-the-counter pain reliever for more than a week, check with your doctor, who can help you find alternatives.

There are preventive prescription medications available for both migraine and tension-type headaches. Factors to consider before trying them include how frequent and debilitating your child's headaches are, and whether or not she is responding to other efforts to prevent and control them. Preventive medications for tension headaches involve daily doses of an anti-inflammatory drug such as ibuprofen or naproxen. For migraines, preventive medicines focus on changing the blood pressure, so they have side effects such as drowsiness. For this reason, some doctors prefer to use prescription medicines, rather than preventive medications, to treat migraine from the outset.

Treating Tension

If your child's headache is tension-type, you'll also want to work on the underlying cause, which is usually stress of some sort. Your first step, according to doctors, is to look for conflict at home or at school, or some event that might be bringing tension into your child's life.

> To reduce the incidence and severity of tension headaches, help your child learn to recognize and express his or her emotions—especially negative ones. Reduce the likelihood of stress buildup by having an atmosphere in your house where you can talk with your child. This might mean sitting down to at least one meal a day together, or taking walks together, or doing other things together that give you time with your child when you can talk. Give your child the message that it's okay to talk about feelings.
>
> —Lonnie Zelter, M.D.,
> Mattel Children's Hospital at UCLA

If you can help your child eliminate the cause of the stress (internal or external), then you can probably prevent future headaches. If the stress is coming from conflict in the home, be extra careful about things like arguing in front of your child. Sometimes, however, the tension comes from school issues.

Often kids who are bright overachievers, but have a hidden learning disability they are working to compensate for, get tension headaches. They can also happen to kids with low-level social anxiety who have problems making friends or dealing with social situations at school. These are kids who are otherwise doing well in school and should like it but don't.

Parents need to be able to recognize the normal stressors and try to take care of those. However, don't keep asking your child "Is your head hurting?" The best way to turn off pain signals is through distraction. Your child might have come up with a self-coping mechanism, such as playing a video game, that is taking his mind off the pain. Your asking only calls his attention back to the pain again. Remember that muscle-tension headaches will not damage children, so there is no harm in letting your child deal with them if he can do so successfully.

—Lonnie Zelter, M.D.,
Mattel Children's Hospital at UCLA

In older children and adolescents, tension headaches are especially common at periods of developmental transition. This could mean when they move from grammar school to junior high, or from junior high to high school. Things like a move to a new school, or trouble in the family, can also contribute. No matter what the cause, doctors say that talking it out is a big help. There are also some other things you can do.

First see if you can massage the head, neck, and shoulders to try and relax the muscles. Circular motions with firm pressure with the fingertips seems to work best, increasing the circulation and loosening the muscles. Your child will let you know what feels good and what doesn't, and you should go with what she wants.

—LONNIE ZELTER, M.D.,
MATTEL CHILDREN'S HOSPITAL AT UCLA

If the headache is tension-type, you can put a warm pack on the muscles to relax them. You can also try other stress-reduction techniques.

—JEROME ESSER, M.D.,
CHILDREN'S HOSPITAL OF WISCONSIN

If you can't figure out the cause of your child's stress, or if it is not easily resolved, you might want to try some alternative techniques. Studies have proved that biofeedback and hypnosis are very effective against both migraine and tension-type headaches. Yoga and acupuncture can also help your child reduce tension and lessen the incidence of headaches.

PRIMARY HEADACHE DISORDER

If your child's headaches are severe and happen often, it's possible that he has primary headache disorder. There are more than 150 types of headaches, according to the American Council for Headache Education. But all of these, if recurrent or chronic, are now treated in much the same way. These headaches can be tension–type, migraine, or combinations of these along with other types of headache. Rather than trying to isolate the specific type of headache, says Siegfried Schmidt, M.D., Ph.D., F.A.F.P., of the University of Florida College of Medicine, doctors have taken to defining and treating the disorder as a whole.

Technically, headaches are chronic if they happen more often than fifteen days per month for more than six months. However, some doctors say that it is just as important to consider how debilitating the headaches are to the child. Is the child having them several times a week? Are they so bad (as is often the case with migraines) that the child can't function?

> If your child has primary headache disorder, it is important that you talk to him and explain what he might feel, and that he isn't a bad person or very ill because he has headaches. Explain that these things are genetically influenced, and that they are often set off by a trigger. Put guilt aside, and realize that some people are just born this way.
>
> —Siegfried Schmidt, M.D., Ph.D., F.A.F.P.,
> University of Florida College of Medicine

If your child is diagnosed with primary headache disorder, your first step is to educate yourself and your family about the headaches. Find a doctor who can help and can work with you. She should be able to offer information about the headaches themselves, as well as ways to manage and treat them. When primary headache disorder is treated appropriately, the patient can lead a normal life. It is important that your child understands this.

You should also talk to your child's teacher and explain about primary headache disorder. Make it clear that you are working on treating the problem but that it might take some time. The teacher might think that your child is pretending to be ill to get out of class or homework, but the type of kids who get primary headache disorder usually aren't like that. These are smart kids and achievers.

> When your child has a headache, teach her to set priorities. Have her plan to do the important stuff first, and

then do the rest as she can, because she might not be able to get everything done. If the important stuff is done first, this means less pressure and stress.

—SIEGFRIED SCHMIDT, M.D., PH.D., F.A.F.P.,
UNIVERSITY OF FLORIDA COLLEGE OF MEDICINE

Keep in mind that for children who have headaches often, they can be as frustrating as they are painful. Don't deny that your child really is in pain, and that the condition can have an emotional and social impact. He might not be able to go to concerts because of the noise, or sleepovers because of the lack of sleep. Help him find ways to cope, and other things he can do to make up for the missed activities.

Though all headaches are real, most don't have a cause that will show up on a brain scan or MRI [Magnetic Resonance Imaging, a noninvasive scan that produces pictures of the inside of the body]. Continuing to look just creates more stress and can make the problem worse. It's probably a better idea to ask your pediatrician to examine your child's neck and shoulders for trigger points that would indicate muscle tension and muscle spasms.

—LONNIE ZELTER, M.D.,
MATTEL CHILDREN'S HOSPITAL AT UCLA

On the Trigger

In order to get your child's recurrent headaches under control, you'll need to make the appropriate lifestyle adjustments. In many cases, this means learning to avoid the triggers that set off the headaches. Some kids are more sensitive to odors or perfumes, others to visual triggers like computers or TV. There's an amazing amount of sensory stimulation in the world today: Television bombards us with an amazing number of images every minute, in addition to video games and computers, music and perfumes.

Triggers can include:

- Foods high in nitrates, such as hot dogs or processed meats
- Chocolate
- Cola and diet cola
- MSG and other preservatives, found in many pre-packaged foods and often in Chinese food
- Cheddar cheese
- Peanut butter or peanuts
- Perfumes
- Cigarette smoke
- Lack of sleep
- Excess sleep
- Skipping meals

The easiest way to tell if any of the major food triggers are causing your child's headaches is to eliminate all of them from the diet for a while, then reintroduce them one at a time. If your child dislikes school lunches, or if you have a teen who is trying to lose weight, do your best to make sure that he isn't skipping meals.

Food additives are the biggest triggers for migraine. Avoid caffeinated foods, things containing MSG, sulfites, and other preservatives. This might mean some canned and pickled foods, and also some processed meats. Parents of children prone to migraine should keep a food diary to help them identify triggers.

—JEROME ESSER, M.D.,
CHILDREN'S HOSPITAL OF WISCONSIN

You should also watch your child's sleep patterns. Many kids get headaches during the summer, when they are allowed to stay up later then go to summer camp the next day, or do something else very active out in the bright sun. Headaches can also be triggered when a child attends a sleepover and stays up all night, then sleeps most of the next afternoon.

Weather changes and hormonal changes (such as those brought on by menstruation) can be triggers as well. These are mainly migraine triggers but can cause tension headaches, too.

> If your child can't eat particular foods because they are headache triggers, it might be easier for him to explain as a food allergy. This can help with peer pressure.
> —SIEGFRIED SCHMIDT, M.D., PH.D., F.A.F.P.,
> UNIVERSITY OF FLORIDA COLLEGE OF MEDICINE

Any lifestyle changes you have to make to manage your child's headaches—whether they involve avoiding certain foods, skipping sleepovers, or watching how much time he spends in the sun or at the computer—can be frustrating for him. Tell him he has a brain that is just more sensitive than anyone else's, so he has to protect it. Sometimes this makes children feel good, and it sounds much better than talking about a "disorder" or an "illness."

Headache Diaries

If you're trying to identify triggers of your child's headaches, many doctors recommend that you help her keep a headache calendar or diary. This will help you and your child's doctor determine whether the headaches happen in response to certain foods or activities.

> Record the start and end time of each headache, and record everything your child ate for twelve hours before the headache and what you did to treat it.

(continued)

This will help you learn about the frequency of headaches your child has, and what might be triggering them.
            —POORVI PATEL, M.D.,
                ST. JOSEPH'S CHILDREN'S HOSPITAL,
                NEW JERSEY

Your doctor will want to know if there is a family history of headache, if there are certain times of the day when your child is most likely to have a headache, and what types of things make the headache better: Tylenol? Sleep? A cold compress?

Not all doctors love the idea of a headache diary, however:

Asking your child to keep a headache diary just calls attention to the pain, because you're asking him to be constantly monitoring his body looking for signs of pain. Kids who keep diaries often have more pain when they're keeping them than when they aren't. Diaries are only useful if the parent has come to believe that the child has headaches all the time. The diary might be able to show that there are actually times when the child is pain-free.
            —LONNIE ZELTER, M.D.,
                MATTEL CHILDREN'S HOSPITAL AT UCLA

Some doctors say that focusing too much time and energy on your child's headache problem is bad for her self-esteem and can actually create tension that makes the problem worse. So even if you're the one keeping a headache diary, don't spend all your time "monitoring" and evaluating your child. She will let you know if she's in pain.

WHEN TO CALL THE DOCTOR

If your child is having problems with headache, there are two main reasons to call the doctor. The first is if there are signs that the headache might be of the "secondary" type—those caused by disease, tumor, or aneurysm. Call your doctor right away if your child has a headache that is extremely severe and sudden, or if you have a child under age five who has recurrent headaches. Also call if your child has headaches that wake her up, if they're getting more frequent or more severe, or if your child experiences morning vomiting with headaches.

Other red flags include headaches that cause balance, motor, or vision problems or loss of consciousness, or headaches that *always* appear on the same side. (It's okay if a person *usually* gets headaches on the same side.) Headache that coincides with high fever and/or stiff neck could be a sign of meningitis, a serious illness that requires immediate medical treatment. Headaches that appear within forty-eight to seventy-two hours after a head injury could be signs of concussion.

> If you're ever worried about your child's headache, go ahead and call the doctor. Getting some information and guidance is better than letting your anxiety build to the point where you pass it on to your child.
>
> —LONNIE ZELTER, M.D.,
> MATTEL CHILDREN'S HOSPITAL AT UCLA

Another reason to call the doctor is if your child's recurrent headaches are disrupting her life. If she is having headaches for a period of three to four weeks without any other illness, or has headaches that are severe enough to miss school without any other illness, she should be evaluated by a pediatrician. If your child has headaches over a long period of time, it isn't likely to be something very serious. If something is really wrong, such as a tumor or aneurysm, it comes on and gets worse fairly quickly.

Be aware that a doctor evaluating your child's headache will often order an MRI or some other imaging test. This doesn't mean that anything is seriously wrong. The doctor is just doing it to help rule out the rare possibility that there is something wrong. So don't panic.

Helpful Websites and Organizations

- **The National Headache Foundation,**
  www.headaches.org, (888) NHF-5552: Offers links
  to support groups and information about the latest
  headache treatments and research. The website
  includes guides to children's headache management
  for both kids and their parents.
- **Headache Care Network for Primary Care,**
  www.headachecare.com: Includes a huge set of
  research articles from a number of credible sources,
  a listing by area of physicians trained in headache
  management, an interactive self-evaluation guide,
  information on prevention and treatment, and a
  chance to chat with other headache sufferers.
- **The American Council for Headache Education,**
  www.achenet.org: Offers discussion and support
  groups, a mailing list, a physician finder, and an
  entire section on kids and headache that includes a
  large list of migraine triggers.

Head Lice

I f your head itches as you read this chapter title, you probably have had a child with head lice. These tiny pests are at the top of every parents' Most Unwanted list, because they are contagious and tough to get rid of, and because many people associate them with poor hygiene. The fact that doctors assert that even the most meticulously clean child can get head lice doesn't make it any easier when that meticulously clean child belongs to you.

Head lice are parasites that live in the hair and feed on blood that they suck from the scalp. They are about 1/10 of an inch in size, and their eggs—often called "nits"—are about the size of a grain of sand. Children most often get infested with lice through direct, head-to-head contact, though lice also can and do spread via hats and combs. Contrary to popular belief, lice do not have wings or powerful legs, so they are incapable of jumping or flying from one head to another, or from an object onto your child's head.

FIRST RESPONSE

SHAMPOO AND CONQUER

While it is possible to rid your child of lice by combing and picking out all live lice and eggs each day, doctors say that most families don't have the time or patience to do this properly. Using this technique means spending an hour or two each day for at least 10 days scrutinizing, combing, and picking your child's hair, and cutting individual eggs out of the hair with a small pair of scissors or pulling the nits down the hair shaft with the fingernails.

Since most children can't sit still for this even if their parents can, doctors say that if your child has an active infestation of lice, your best course of action is to treat everyone in the family who has lice with a medicated shampoo or cream rinse. The most popular of these are Nix, a cream rinse with a one-percent solution of permethrin, and Rid, a medicated shampoo containing pyrethrins. Both are available over the counter.

> My first-line recommendation is Nix. There is resistance among lice to all medications, but there seems to be less resistance to Nix. If this treatment fails, the lice are either resistant to Nix, or you did it wrong.
>
> —DANIEL KROWCHUCK, M.D.,
> BRENNER CHILDREN'S HOSPITAL,
> WINSTON-SALEM, NORTH CAROLINA

COMFORT CARE

THE CREAM RINSE

Many parents who use medicated shampoos and cream rinses find them to be ineffective. There are two possible reasons for this. The first, and doctors say most common, is that parents make some mistake and use the product improperly.

> Before using the Nix cream rinse, first shampoo the hair with a dish-washing detergent (not the type you use in the dishwasher, but the type you use to wash dishes by hand). The brand Dawn works best. It helps detach the "cement" that holds the lice eggs to the hair shaft.
> —BARBARA ZIOGAS KAYE, M.D.,
> JOHN DEMPSEY HOSPITAL,
> FARMINGTON, CONNECTICUT

Many parents, for instance, put the cream rinse on while the hair is still dripping wet, and the water dilutes the medication to the point where it won't kill the lice. Instead, after washing your child's hair, you should pat it as dry as possible with a towel, leaving it only a little damp. (Wash the towel in very hot water afterward.)

Don't put a regular conditioner on the hair before using a medicated shampoo or cream rinse, as the oils in the conditioner will keep the medication from binding properly to the hair.

Another mistake parents make—especially if they are trying to treat more than one person with a single bottle of cream rinse—is to put too little of the product on the hair. You should use the full amount suggested on the packaging, and make sure that your child's hair is covered with the rinse from scalp to ends. Skimping will leave patches of unmedicated hair where lice can survive.

Since the products contain pesticides, many parents are uncomfortable using them and don't leave them on long enough. However, rinsing the product out before the full ten minutes (measured by the clock) recommended on the package will just mean that the lice aren't killed, and you will end up treating your child again and again.

THE COMB-OUT

Because the medicated shampoos and conditioners—despite what it might say on the package—might not kill all of the lice, you'll still have to comb your child's hair to pick up any lice the products missed. The comb will *not,* as many people believe, remove the eggs, says Dr. Krowchuck, because the eggs are cemented to the hair shaft and are not likely to come off in the comb.

Choose a sturdy, fine-toothed comb designed for lice removal, and comb section by section in an orderly fashion. Krowchuck recommends combing for the first time right after treatment, while the hair is still wet, while Barbara Ziogas Kaye, M.D., of John Dempsey Hospital, says that waiting until the next morning when the hair is dry makes combing easier.

Either way, it is best to comb section by section in an orderly fashion, and section off longer hair with barrettes or clips to make it more manageable.

You don't need to look for lice while you comb, so you don't need to spend lots of time scrutinizing the hair. You'll be able to see the live lice when you get them on the comb. Just concentrate on combing the hair correctly and covering every section of the head from scalp to end. This makes the combing go much more quickly for your child.

—DANIEL KROWCHUCK, M.D.,
BRENNER CHILDREN'S HOSPITAL,
WINSTON-SALEM, NORTH CAROLINA

You may find live lice on your child's head if you comb right after treatment. Pick them off the comb with a tissue and flush them down the toilet. However, if you wait until the morning after treatment to comb, any lice you find should be dead. If you find live lice at this point and you did the treatment correctly, the lice are resistant to the medication.

Re-treat the hair a week to ten days after the first treatment, to kill any newly hatched lice. Since the cream rinse won't necessarily kill all of the eggs, this is an essential step.

> Don't re-treat too early. Newly hatched lice do not have a central nervous system for the first four days of life, and so will not be susceptible to the medications, which attack the central nervous system.
>
> —DANIEL KROWCHUCK, M.D.,
> BRENNER CHILDREN'S HOSPITAL,
> WINSTON-SALEM, NORTH CAROLINA

Comb the hair a couple of times per week between treatments. You don't have to do it every day, but do it at least once, midway between treatments. Picking out any new lice that hatch between treatments will help keep a new population of lice from getting started. After the second treatment with medicated shampoo or cream rinse, comb your child's hair at least one more time in case any lice have survived.

Some parents find that combing doesn't work. They pull the nits down the hairshaft and dispose of them in alcohol. If this route works for you, you might try sitting the child in front of a favorite video. Positioning a very bright light on the child's scalp will help you spot the tiny nits.

TREATING THE HOUSE

Because there is some chance that lice will spread via combs, clothes, bedding, or furniture, doctors recommend that you take measures to eliminate any stray lice in your home. This is important, but not as important as killing all of the lice on everyone's heads, says Dr. Kaye. Lice die within fifty-five hours away from their host, so they can't live very long on brushes, combs, furniture, or other things.

> Soak combs, brushes, and hair accessories for ten minutes in a dish of warm water to which you've added a little Nix.
>
> —BARBARA ZIOGAS KAYE, M.D.,
> JOHN DEMPSEY HOSPITAL,
> FARMINGTON, CONNECTICUT

To treat the home, change your child's bedding after each treatment with medicated shampoo or cream rinse. Wash or dry clean all bedding, clothing, hats, and coats. Bag stuffed animals that can't be washed in plastic with a tight seal, for three days to two weeks, until any lice hiding there are dead.

Vacuum other areas that could harbor lice, such as mattresses, carpets, or the upper part of the back of your sofa, and throw the vacuum cleaner bag away afterward just to be safe.

THE RE-CHECK

Doctors say that sometimes parents think a lice treatment has failed when it has not. The parent has just mistaken dead eggs or empty egg casings, aphids, or other insects, pieces of hair shaft, or even dandruff for a lice infestation.

Even eggs or egg casings aren't cause for concern if they are far from the scalp. Lice generally attach their eggs within half an inch of the scalp. Eggs found farther from the scalp than that have been there long enough for the hair to have grown and are probably either already hatched or dead.

At this point, your child is probably used to scratching his head, and asking him if his head itches will probably give him the urge to scratch. Rather than asking, watch discreetly to see if he scratches.

—DANIEL KROWCHUCK, M.D.,
BRENNER CHILDREN'S HOSPITAL,
WINSTON-SALEM, NORTH CAROLINA

If you really believe you're having repeated episodes of lice, it is a good idea to see the doctor to make sure that what you're seeing is an active infestation, and not one of these other things. Try blowing on the suspect area. If the particle blows away, it's probably dandruff.

Sure signs of lice infestation include live lice on the scalp or hair, eggs attached very close to the scalp (within ½ inch), and active itching.

OTHER THINGS TO TRY

Nonprescription alternatives to the medicated shampoo and cream rinse route all seem to involve smothering the lice with some sort of oil. Both Kaye and Krowchuck recommend Hair Clear 123, a difficult to find product that contains a mixture of organic oils. It hasn't been studied rigorously, but is nontoxic and has been effective for some people.

I have had at least one patient get rid of her child's lice by putting Vaseline on his hair, but she said it was actually just as bad as dealing with the lice. Vaseline is extremely difficult to get out of the hair. To remove it, you have to cover it with talcum powder and then comb out as much as you can. Then you have to wash the hair with dish-washing liquid.

—BARBARA ZIOGAS KAYE, M.D.,
JOHN DEMPSEY HOSPITAL,
FARMINGTON, CONNECTICUT

You can also try putting full-fat mayonnaise on the scalp and leaving it on overnight under a shower cap to smother the lice.

Never put gasoline or other types of insecticides (such as those made for your yard or home) on your child's head. This could be a fatal mistake.

WHEN TO CALL THE DOCTOR

If your child has resistant head lice, there are several options for treatment. Most of these involve calling your doctor, as they are only available by prescription. Lindane and Kwell were once popular prescription treatments for lice, but now most doctors recommend against them because of concerns about toxicity.

Instead, they prefer Ovid, a malathion preparation that appears to be highly effective. It kills quickly, but must be used with great care because it is flammable. If you are using Ovid, you cannot dry your child's hair with a blow dryer or smoke around your child. Bactrim, an oral antibiotic, can disrupt the digestion or reproductive systems of lice and might also be helpful.

You might not be thrilled about the idea of using lice-specific pesticides on your child's head, but if used correctly, doctors insist that they are safe. And since they are generally effective in one treatment, your child's exposure will be minimal.

Insect Stings or Bites

If your child likes to spend time outdoors, he's likely to suffer a few insect stings and bites. Doctors report that mosquitoes, bees—including honeybees, bumblebees, hornets, and wasps—ticks, spiders, fleas, and ants are the most likely crawling creatures waiting to sink teeth or stinger into your little one.

A few of these stings or bites can be serious or even fatal. Some can cause a severe allergic reaction. Most, however, won't cause more than some pain, swelling, and itch.

FIRST RESPONSE

FIND THE BITER

If your child comes to you with a bite or sting, first remove her from the area where she was stung, in case there are more bugs nearby. Next, try to find out what stung her. Look for the stinger, bumps or welts, or the bugs themselves. Remove any bugs that are present, so they don't sting again.

If you suspect that your child was bitten by either of the two main types of poisonous spiders common in North America—the black widow and the brown recluse—call your doctor immediately. Spider bites are rare but can be serious.

Also seek medical attention if your child shows signs of severe allergic reaction (see page 21). Otherwise, you can just apply the appropriate comfort-care measures at home.

Doctors advise that children who have had severe allergic reactions to insect bites or stings—especially reactions involving respiratory distress—should have an Epi-Pen available at all times. These devices allow an adult, or even an older child, to give an injection of epinephrine, which will keep the airways open.

COMFORT CARE

Unless you need to seek medical attention for an allergic reaction, you can treat most insect bites and stings at home by removing the stinger or insect and taking measures to ease pain, swelling, and itch. It's also a good idea to prevent bites and stings if your children will be outdoors.

STINGERS AND TICKS

If your child is bitten by a tick or stung by a bee, you'll be faced with the tricky task of removing the bug or stinger from your child's skin without making matters worse. If you go about this the wrong way, you could end up squeezing more venom or other irritating material into the skin, or leaving a piece of the tick behind.

To remove a tick, hold the head with tweezers and avoid squeezing the body, or you're likely to squeeze material into your child's skin and create infection.

—ANWAR AL-HADDAWI, M.D.,
ST. JOSEPH'S CHILDREN'S HOSPITAL, NEW JERSEY

Doctors recommend using tweezers for ticks and pulling straight back, rather than twisting, to keep the tick from breaking apart. A tick bite is a serious matter due to the risk of ailments like Rocky Mountain spotted fever or Lyme disease. Your child will need medical attention, and you should bring the tick with you to the doctor.

You should never use a lit match, a cigarette, or alcohol to try to make a tick "back up" on its own. You should also avoid covering the tick with petroleum jelly or nail polish in an attempt to smother it. Matches or cigarettes could injure your child, and these other measures are only likely to make the tick more difficult to remove in the end. If you end up leaving any part of the tick under your child's skin after pulling it out with tweezers, remove the piece using a needle sterilized in alcohol, or held in a flame and wiped clean with a tissue.

Along Came a Spider

According to the Ohio State University Department of Entomology, black widow spiders have shiny, jet-black abdomens marked with two reddish or yellowish triangles that form an hourglass shape. They are about an inch and a half long when the legs are spread, and are considered the most venomous spiders in North America.

The spiders are most often found outdoors in trash or rubble piles, or under and around houses, in sheds and garages. The spiders are shy, won't bite unless disturbed, and are most active at night.

(continued)

The black widow bite often leaves a circular red mark on the skin with a red area around the pale center, says Connie Kostacos, M.D., of Columbia Presbyterian Medical Center. This is called a target mark and might be followed by muscle pain and cramping in the stomach, back, or sides. Sometimes the child is reluctant to walk because of the pain. The bite might also cause chest pain or difficulty breathing.

The brown recluse spider, found mainly in the southern and midwestern states, is yellowish tan to dark brown, with delicate grayish to dark brown legs. It has three pairs of eyes in a semicircle on its head, with a violin-shaped dark marking behind the eyes. The neck of the "violin" points down toward the abdomen. These spiders are most often found in undisturbed areas such as closets, basements, and cellars, or under furniture or carpets. They also live in sheltered corners outdoors, such as sheds or woodpiles. The spiders are not aggressive and generally only bite when touched or disturbed.

The brown recluse bite might cause a minor reaction with mild itching, or a more intense burning sensation that progresses to a blister in the area of the bite, which eventually becomes ulcerated. If the bite is on an area with lots of fatty tissue, these can go quite deep and eventually require plastic surgery. You can also get flulike symptoms from these bites.

If your child was playing in an area where one of these spiders might be—such as around an old woodpile or in the garage—and shows symptoms of a spider bite, clean the area with soap and water and call the doctor. Deaths from spider bites are rare but much more common in small children and the elderly.

Deer ticks are about the size of the head of a pin and are found throughout the United States, but especially in New England and parts of the Midwest. They have been known to carry Lyme disease and ehrlichiosis. Dog ticks are very common throughout the country and can be up to one-half-inch long. They can carry ehrlichiosis, and also Rocky Mountain spotted fever.

Tick-borne diseases have flu-like symptoms such as fever, chills, headache, muscle or joint pain, nausea and vomiting, cough, stomach pain, and sore throat. Your child might also have a rash. Symptoms will probably begin a few days to a week after the tick bite. If caught in the early stages, these diseases are generally not serious and can be treated with antibiotics. However, because the symptoms are often mistaken for flu, many patients don't get medical attention as early as they should. If your child develops flu-like symptoms within a week or two of a tick bite, you should call your doctor right away.

Parents usually squeeze the attached venom sack when they're trying to remove a bee stinger. This expresses more venom into the skin and makes things worse. Instead of pulling or squeezing, scrape the stinger out with clean fingernails or a credit card.
—HELEN SINH-DANG, M.D.,
BOYS TOWN NATIONAL RESEARCH HOSPITAL,
OMAHA, NEBRASKA

Whether you're dealing with a bee sting or a tick, wash the area thoroughly once the bug or stinger is out, and give your child a dose of oral Benadryl to prevent swelling and the mild reaction that often comes in response to a bite or sting.

Meat tenderizer is okay for bee stings if you have it handy. However, it's not worth going out to look for it if you don't. By the time you get back, it will be too late for it to do any good.
—MAUREEN KAYS, M.D.,
SHANDS CHILDREN'S HOSPITAL
AT THE UNIVERSITY OF FLORIDA

In cases of bee sting, doctors also recommend applying ice and elevating the wound to prevent swelling. Meat tenderizer, an old home remedy, has an enzyme that attacks the proteins released in the bee venom, so applying a paste of meat tenderizer can be helpful.

PAIN

Once the insect or stinger is out, you can focus on the pain from the bite or sting. Doctors say that oral Benadryl, over-the-counter pain relievers, and cold compresses will help with both the pain and swelling.

> If your child is bitten or stung and the area is red and painful, ice it. You can also give acetaminophen for pain, or put a topical antiseptic on the bite itself.
>
> —CONNIE KOSTACOS, M.D.,
> COLUMBIA PRESBYTERIAN MEDICAL CENTER

You can make a cold compress by putting some ice in a plastic bag and wrapping it in a wet washcloth, or by just soaking a washcloth in cold water. Avoid rubbing the area, which can cause itch, or spread the venom or infection and damage the skin.

> Use Noxema or some other cold cream and call it "magic cream." Applying this to the bite will be cooling, and it sometimes has a placebo effect.
>
> —MAUREEN KAYS, M.D.,
> SHANDS CHILDREN'S HOSPITAL
> AT THE UNIVERSITY OF FLORIDA

Doctors recommend always having some over-the-counter hydrocortisone cream and oral Benadryl on hand, so they can be used right away in cases of insect bite or sting. However, don't apply hydrocortisone for more than a week without checking with your doctor. In extreme cases it has been known to cause skin problems.

ITCHING

If your child's bite is from a mosquito or ant, you're likely to have a problem with itch—or rather, with convincing your child not to scratch. If your child scratches an insect bite enough to break the skin, it could become infected and eventually require treatment with antibiotics.

> Itch-X is a good over-the-counter medication that helps with mild bites. It's safe, and not absorbed through the skin. Avoid Benadryl creams, as too much is absorbed through the skin. It's also not a good idea to use antibiotic creams unnecessarily, as they help build up antibiotic-resistant strains of bacteria.
>
> —MAUREEN KAYS, M.D.,
> SHANDS CHILDREN'S HOSPITAL
> AT THE UNIVERSITY OF FLORIDA

There are a number of over-the-counter anti-itch medications available, and doctors say that most of them are safe to use. Calamine lotion and hydrocortisone cream seem to be among the favorites.

> When you apply hydrocortisone cream, don't just dab it on. Rub it in well until it is absorbed. This feels good to the child if the bite is itching, but it won't damage the skin like his scratching will. Teach your child to rub itching bites with the soft part of the finger, rather than scratching with the fingernails, or to pinch the bite gently. This will help relieve the itching without damaging the skin.
>
> —HELEN SINH-DANG, M.D.,
> BOYS TOWN NATIONAL RESEARCH HOSPITAL,
> OMAHA, NEBRASKA

Whatever you're planning to use to combat the itch, apply it as soon as you discover the bite, rather than waiting until your child starts to scratch. The scratching tends to make the itch worse, so it's better to nip the itch in the bud and prevent a vicious cycle from beginning.

> If your child is so bothered by an itch that she can't sleep, you can give [oral] Benadryl at night. Avoid topical Caladryl, however, as it causes too much medication to be absorbed by the skin.
> —CONNIE KOSTACOS, M.D.,
> COLUMBIA PRESBYTERIAN MEDICAL CENTER

Call the doctor if your child has fever following an insect bite, or if the area of the bite is warm to the touch, getting bigger, or has red lines radiating from it. These are signs that the area has become infected and needs medical attention.

PREVENTION

When your family is spending time outdoors, think about where your children will be playing, and take some measures to help them avoid insect bites or stings. Avoid dressing your kids in bright fabrics or using products that contain a lot of perfume, as these things will attract insects. Dress the family in long sleeves and long pants, and make sure your kids wear shoes at all times.

> Be aware of what bugs are in your area. Do the mosquitoes or ticks there carry disease? Do you have fire ants? Are there many wasps or bees?
> —MAUREEN KAYS, M.D.,
> SHANDS CHILDREN'S HOSPITAL
> AT THE UNIVERSITY OF FLORIDA

It's best to stay indoors at times when insects are most likely to bite, such as at dusk and dawn for mosquitoes. If you plan to spend lots of time outside in an area where you know there are insects, rub your children down with insect repellent. Just make sure you keep it away from the hands and face.

At home, make sure your pets are free of fleas. Fleas love small children. And keep garbage cans covered at all times, as they attract insects.

Don't use insect repellents with more than a 10 percent concentration of DEET [Diethyltoluamide, the active ingredient] on children. You can use citronella-based repellents that are all-natural as an alternative.

—CONNIE KOSTACOS, M.D.,
COLUMBIA PRESBYTERIAN MEDICAL CENTER

WHEN TO CALL THE DOCTOR

Doctors say the only serious mistake parents make when dealing with an insect bite or sting is not realizing when they should seek medical attention. If you suspect your child has been bitten by a poisonous spider, if insects in your area carry disease, or if your child seems to be having an allergic reaction to an insect bite or sting, seek medical attention.

Signs of systemic allergic reaction—a reaction involving your child's whole body—include widespread rash or hives, drooling, wheezing, chest pain, swelling in the face, tongue, or throat, and difficulty breathing or swallowing. If your child has any of these symptoms following an insect bite or sting, call your doctor or emergency medical services immediately. These reactions can be life-threatening and often require treatment within ten to twenty minutes.

Signs of a local allergic reaction include extreme redness, swelling (especially swelling that goes beyond two inches in diameter), and severe itch at the area of the bite. These aren't generally life-threatening, but they still merit a call to the doctor. Though life-threatening allergic reactions usually don't occur until at least the second bite or sting, a mild allergic reaction is a sign that the next sting might be worse. Consult your doctor, who will decide whether your child should be referred to an allergist or maybe given an Epi-Pen (an epinephrine auto injector) to carry in case of another sting.

Even if your child doesn't have an allergic reaction, you'll need to call if a bite becomes infected from scratching.

Itching Rash

What could be more frustrating than trying to convince a kid with an itch not to scratch? There are any number of irritations, allergies, and fungal infections that can cause itching rashes in kids, and the type your child is most likely to encounter depends on his age.

Kids who are mobile and can get out and into things get different rashes than kids who can't. Mobile kids are most likely to get poison ivy, poison oak, or poison sumac. They can also get contagious rashes such as scabies—a skin infection caused by a parasite—or ringworm, a fungal infection of the skin that has nothing to do with worms. Infants are more likely to get contagious rashes from caregivers or family members than to come in contact with rash-causing plants.

Children of any age can have hives (raised red bumps or welts) or an allergic rash caused by medication or a reaction to jewelry, especially nickel. Illnesses, such as chicken pox (see "Chicken Pox"), can also cause rash. But probably the most common itching rash in kids is atopic dermatitis (eczema). It will strike at least 10 percent of all kids in one form or another during childhood, and is really just severely dry skin.

Contagious Rashes

Most of the more common rashes are not contagious. However, there are a few that are:

- Impetigo: Usually caused by a strep or staph infection, this is a blistered rash with honey-colored secretions that turn into honey-colored crusts.
- Molluscum contagiosum: This viral infection creates big, rounded red pimples, sometimes in groups or clusters.
- Scabies: This is an infestation of the skin by mites similar to lice. It causes red, itchy, swollen lumps, usually at the wrist, armpit, genitals, and buttocks, or between the fingers or toes.
- Poison oak, ivy, or sumac: The rash itself is not contagious. However, the oil from contact with the plant can be passed from one person to another through contact with the skin, clothes, or furniture.

To keep rashes that might be contagious from spreading, don't bathe siblings together or let them share towels, clothes, or hats. Wash your child's clothes separately in hot water and bathe her often. In some cases, you might have to keep her home from school or day care.

FIRST RESPONSE

CONTAIN AND CONQUER

If you're trying to relieve your child's itch, first find out why she's scratching. The most common cause is dry skin, but it could also be an infection, illness, or allergy.

Jewelry, hair dyes, and makeup are common itch culprits. Food allergies make an important contribution to eczema, and eliminating the allergen will almost always make it milder. If your child has been in contact with poison ivy, oak, or sumac, wash the oil from the offending plant off of his skin and clothes right away. If others come in contact with the oil, they'll probably get a rash, too.

If your child has a contagious rash—scabies and head lice are the most contagious—take steps to keep it from spreading to the rest of the family and beyond. If your child has lice, don't share combs, brushes, hats, towels, or clothing. Scabies is extremely difficult to keep from spreading among immediate family members who have close contact, because the parasites easily move from one person to another, but the entire family is generally treated at once. However, your child will probably have to stay home from school until the treatment takes effect.

If the itch is just from dry skin, you can take measures to moisturize, which will stop the itch.

Prickly Heat

Prickly heat, or heat rash, causes tiny red bumps on the neck, groin, armpits, face, and chest. It can occur at any age but is most common in newborns.

It happens when the skin overheats and isn't allowed to breathe. The body sweats, but the sweat is trapped, which

(continued)

causes the rash. The best way to prevent it is to keep your child clean, cool, and dry. Don't overbundle or overheat your child. Dress your baby in lightweight, breathable cotton. Giving warm baths, rather than hot, and using air-conditioning in the summer will help.

A good guideline for making sure you don't overdress your baby is that he should wear one more layer of light clothing than you have on. This might include a light blanket to keep the sun off.

—JILL REEL, M.D.,
BOYS TOWN NATIONAL RESEARCH HOSPITAL,
OMAHA, NEBRASKA

If the rash itches, you can treat it with over-the-counter hydrocortisone cream. However, try not to use a lot of moisturizing lotion, which can make the rash worse. The rash should resolve in a few days, as long as your child stays cool and dry and doesn't become overheated again.

Call the doctor if your child is acting fussy, has a fever, or is not eating or sleeping well. Also call if the rash looks blistered or weeping or shows other signs of infection.

COMFORT CARE

Stopping the itch caused by your child's rash will make your child feel better and give the rash time to heal. In most cases, this is as simple as keeping the skin well hydrated and using an over-the-counter medication.

FIGHTING DRY SKIN

One of the most common reasons for children to have an itching rash is dry skin, which in its most serious form is called eczema. To combat dry skin, doctors recommend that you do two things: First, avoid drying out your child's skin; second, use moisturizers to keep the skin hydrated.

The water (moisture) is held in your skin by a layer of oil. Soaps dissolve that layer of oil and let the water evaporate out of the skin. So the most common mistake is using too much soap and overcleaning the skin. Doctors recommend using the least amount of soap possible and lots of water.

Bathe your child with a minimal amount of soap, then rinse all the soap away down the drain, fill the tub with clean water, and let your child play there to hydrate the skin. Instead of bubble bath, use bath oil, which leaves an oil slick on the surface of the water and then on the surface of the skin. This holds the water in the skin.

—MELVIN BERGER, M.D., PH.D.,
RAINBOW BABIES AND CHILDREN'S HOSPITAL,
CLEVELAND, OHIO

If you're putting your child in the tub and shampooing her hair first, then letting her play, the shampoo in the water counts as bubble bath. If you're going to use it, you need to make sure that you slather your child with a good moisturizer right after the bath to keep moisture in the skin.

—JAMES G.H. DINULOS, M.D.,
CHILDREN'S HOSPITAL AT DARTMOUTH

Doctors warn against using bubble bath if your child has dry skin, because in a tub full of bubbles, your child is basically soaking in soap. After the bath, doctors recommend that you let the skin air-dry thoroughly, or pat it dry gently. Vigorous rubbing—even though it might feel good to a child who is itchy—can irritate the skin. "Don't let them use the towel like a giant scratching post," advises Melvin Berger, M.D., Ph.D., and chief of allergy and immunology at Rainbow Babies and Children's Hospital.

Don't limit baths if your child has eczema or an itch due to dry skin. Give a short bath and use lotion within five minutes of drying the skin. The bath hydrates the skin, and the lotion holds in the moisture. Oatmeal baths are also good for itch. Make the water warm, not hot, and limit the bath to five to ten minutes.

—LISA GELLES, M.D.,
THE CHILDREN'S MEDICAL CENTER OF DAYTON

Doctors generally advise using a heavy cream rather than a light lotion, as the heavier creams are better at trapping moisture. Many doctors say that plain petroleum jelly is an excellent and inexpensive moisturizer.

Moisturize, moisturize, moisturize. To do this properly, you need to use a heavy cream with water beaten into it. Creams from a jar rather than a bottle tend to be heavier. Look for the word "emollient" on the label. Some good brand names are Eucerin and Aquaphore. Lubriderm is also okay.

—MELVIN BERGER, M.D., PH.D.,
RAINBOW BABIES AND CHILDREN'S HOSPITAL

Dry air—from heating or air-conditioning, or in a dry climate—can also rob moisture from the skin. Keep an eye on the humidity level in your home, and make sure there is plenty of moisture in the air.

Use a cool-mist humidifier at night during the dry months, or if your air-conditioning or heating system is drying out the air in the house, to keep the skin moist.

—JILL REEL, M.D.,
BOYS TOWN NATIONAL RESEARCH HOSPITAL,
OMAHA, NEBRASKA

OTHER ITCH STOPPERS

There are plenty of reasons to keep your child from scratching. The most important is that if your child scratches enough to break the skin, it can cause infection and scarring. Your child is especially vulnerable to infections such as impetigo, staph, and strep if he has a cold or runny nose along with the itchy rash, because bacteria that gets on the hands from wiping or blowing the nose can be scratched into the skin.

> To help minimize the damage from scratching, keep your child's fingernails cut short. Calamine lotion can help dry up cases of poison ivy or poison oak, as can baking-soda baths. However, don't use them for eczema, where the itching is caused by dry skin.
> —JILL REEL, M.D.,
> BOYS TOWN NATIONAL RESEARCH HOSPITAL,
> OMAHA, NEBRASKA

The scratching also irritates your child's already irritated skin and can actually make a mild rash worse. This is especially true if your child has eczema, where there is an itch-scratch-itch cycle. The more she scratches, the more she will itch.

> During the day, provide distractions to help keep your child from scratching. A lot of kids scratch while they're sitting and watching TV. If they're active, they're less likely to scratch. If the itching is from dry skin, you can let them help you apply moisturizer to help keep them busy. At night, put them in long-sleeved pajamas with long pants if weather permits.
> —LISA GELLES, M.D.,
> THE CHILDREN'S MEDICAL CENTER OF DAYTON

To help stop the itching, try oral medications or topical creams. Over-the-counter antihistamines such as Benadryl can be a big help. These make some kids sleepy, but in others they have the opposite effect. Try a dose during a day when your child will be at home: If it makes her sleepy, use it at night, but avoid it if it keeps your child awake. You can also get long-acting, nonsedating antihistamines with a doctor's prescription.

> Be careful about using antibiotic creams on rashes. These are sensitizing and could cause an allergy to the medication in the cream, especially if used on broken skin. Don't use these on eczema unless you talk to your doctor first. Your doctor might prefer to give you a prescription antibiotic cream using ingredients that are less sensitizing.
> —MELVIN BERGER, M.D., PH.D.,
> RAINBOW BABIES AND CHILDREN'S HOSPITAL

Doctors also warn against using topical antihistamines such as Benadryl cream, however, because they allow too much medication to be absorbed through the skin and could cause your child to develop an allergy. Over-the-counter hydrocortisone creams are good, and generally aren't strong enough to do any harm, but parents should be careful. If you're going to use them for an extended period of time, or around the face, talk to your doctor first.

WHEN TO CALL THE DOCTOR

If your child develops hives following a dose of medication or an insect bite or sting (See "Insect Bites or Stings"), call the doctor immediately, especially if your child is wheezing or having trouble breathing. This could mean that your child is having a life-threatening allergic reaction.

If the rash is spreading or infecting other members of the family, it is likely contagious and will need medical treatment. Also call the doctor if your child has fever or other symptoms, which are signs that your child's rash is being caused by an illness. This is especially true if your child has purplish hives along with fever and stiff neck. These are signs of meningitis.

Even if your child has a less serious rash, contact your doctor if it is widespread and making your child so uncomfortable that she can't sleep or take part in normal daily activities. If your child's rash is on the face or involves the eye, or if it shows signs of infection—yellow crusting, redness, swelling, odor, weeping, tenderness, or increased warmth—a doctor should look at it. Finally, any rash that doesn't start to improve after one or two days of treatment with hydrocortisone cream merits medical attention.

Rash Reconnaissance

Before you call your doctor about your child's rash, do some investigating and have the following information ready:

- Does your child have any underlying medical conditions or allergies?
- Is your child taking any medication?
- Has your child had any recent illnesses?
- Has your child come in contact with anyone who might have infected her? Is there an outbreak of rash at your child's school or day-care center?
- Does anyone else in the family have the rash?
- Do you have pets?

(continued)

- Was your child bitten or stung by a bee or other insect?
- Has your child been eating anything she usually doesn't eat?
- Was your child playing outdoors?
- How long has the rash been there?
- What measures have you taken to try and treat the rash?
- Is there anything you have found that makes the rash worse?
- Does your child have a fever?
- Does your child have any complaints affecting the entire body, such as headache, nausea, or upset stomach?
- Is your child scratching at night? During the day?
- Is your child's activity level normal?

Muscle Ache

Most people think about muscle pain in terms of adult athletes or the elderly, not as something we imagine happening to children. However, many things can make a child's muscles ache. You get very few complaints of pain in very young children, but that doesn't mean they don't have it. They just don't talk about it.

Younger kids are most likely to have aching muscles because of the flu or another illness with fever. As kids approach middle childhood, "growing pains"—middle-of-the-night leg pains—are likely to be a factor. Active and athletic kids might also have complaints because of overuse, similar to that of adults.

FIRST RESPONSE

THE DOSE WITH THE MOST

If your child complains of muscle ache, start with a dose of over-the-counter medication. Doctors recommend both acetaminophen and ibuprofen for children with muscle pain; some say that acetaminophen—found in Tylenol—is best because it is gentler on the stomach. Others find that ibuprofen—found in Motrin and Advil—is more effective in kids four and older because it has an anti-inflammatory agent as well as a pain reliever.

Avoid giving aspirin to children, except under the advice of a doctor—especially if your child has muscle ache that you suspect is caused by flu or another virus—because of the danger of Reye's syndrome, a potentially fatal complication.

COMFORT CARE

If your child's muscle pain is from an illness, it should go away once your child is better. Doing your best to help resolve the illness will help. If the pain is from growing, or playing too hard, you can most likely help make your child feel better at home with simple things such as rest, ice, massage, and reassurance.

GROWING PAINS

Between the ages of two and eight, it's not uncommon for children to have growing pains. These are leg pains or cramps that generally happen in the middle of the night, on the front of one or both legs. There's no swelling or redness, and the pain is always gone in the morning.

Warm baths, heating pads, acetaminophen or ibupro-
fen, stretching, or massage will sometimes help.
— KATHRYN MCLEOD, M.D.,
MEDICAL COLLEGE OF GEORGIA

If your child still has pain in the morning, it's probably
not from growing pains. No one is certain what causes them.
Some doctors speculate that they might be caused by the
stretching and pulling of the muscles and tendons during
periods of rapid growth. Others say that growing has nothing
to do with it.

If your child always complains about pain in one specific
location, or seems to have pain that also comes during
the day, or doesn't respond to Tylenol, seek medical
attention. This is something more than growing pains.
— DAVID ROYE, M.D.,
CHILDREN'S HOSPITAL OF NEW YORK

PLAYING PAINS

Believe it or not, kids can overdo it just like adults. So if your
child has been working extra hard for the team, or even doing
something like yard work, he can end up sore the next day,
the same way you might. Treatment for these aches and pains,
which doctors call "overuse injuries," is fairly simple, and
there's lots you can do to prevent them from happening again.

Treatment

If you have a young athlete in the family, you should remember your RICE. The acronym stands for rest, ice, compression, and elevation, and it's standard first aid for aching
muscles. Start with some ice cubes in a plastic bag, wrapped
in a towel, which doctors say is both effective and reassuring

to your child. Ice the area periodically (ten or twenty minutes at a time, a few times a day) for the first twelve to twenty-four hours. (After that, icing won't help.)

> Avoid using things like Ben-Gay, which can be absorbed through the skin. When you're rubbing something onto a child's skin, because they are smaller than adults, you're actually rubbing it onto a much greater surface area of the body than with an adult. The skin can absorb too much, and the child can either become overdosed or become sensitive to the ingredients in the medication.
> —MAUREEN KAYS, M.D.,
> SHANDS HOSPITAL, UNIVERSITY OF FLORIDA

If it's convenient, wrap the area in a bandage and keep it elevated as much as possible to minimize the swelling. This works even for sore muscles in the upper extremities. You don't have to prop the injured area up too far. It just needs to be at or above the level of the heart.

After a day or two, when the swelling should be down, doctors recommend switching to warm baths, heat packs, and gentle massage to relax and loosen up the sore muscles. However, if the pain is from a trauma with bruising (see "Bruises and Black Eyes") avoid heat and continue with the ice.

If your child is having pain due to exercise, back off her activity level for a while. Once the pain is gone, have her start slow and gradually work back up to her normal range of activity.

Prevention

Preventing sports injuries is, of course, much better than treating them. And the place to start, according to doctors, is by making sure your child is active and in reasonable shape. Just simple outdoor play is great exercise for kids and something many will do eagerly (or with minimal encourage-

What's That Bump?

If your child develops painful swelling on the "bump" just below the kneecap, he could have Osgood-Schlatter disease, which isn't actually a disease at all. It is a type of overuse injury—most common in kids around the age of ten—that occurs because the limb is still growing.

You can treat it with rest and ice, just like most other sports injuries. Once the initial pain and swelling are gone, ibuprofen before sports activities will prevent further pain and swelling and allow your child to stay in the game. The condition almost always resolves itself on its own without complications, but you should see your pediatrician if you are concerned or if your child is in a great deal of pain.

ment). All you have to do is shut off the Nintendo and the computer and get them outside to play.

> Younger kids, unless they are being pushed, will usually stop physical activity if it hurts them. Older kids, however, might push themselves if they are in a competitive situation. If you think this might be happening to your child and it's causing pain, talk to the coach.
>
> —MAUREEN KAYS, M.D.,
> SHANDS HOSPITAL, UNIVERSITY OF FLORIDA

If your child is involved in sports, or if you are trying to involve her, let her choose her own activities. This will help ensure that what your child is doing is fun and age-appropriate. If your sports kid is complaining of pain, make sure that he's okay from a psychosocial standpoint. Sometimes a child is afraid to tell his parents that he doesn't like a particular sport, or being on a particular team, and complaining of pain is an easy way out.

If your child is involved in sports, it's important for you to watch and pay attention to her performance. Children often don't complain of pain, so if you see that the way they walk or run, or anything else about their performance, changes, you should suspect that something is wrong.

—DAVID ROYE, M.D,
CHILDREN'S HOSPITAL OF NEW YORK

Make sure that your child's equipment—especially the shoes—is good. Don't skimp on shoes, even if they are expensive. If your child is a runner, make sure he trains on soft surfaces as much as possible.

—KATHRYN MCLEOD, M.D.,
MEDICAL COLLEGE OF GEORGIA

Parents must also remember that children are not little adults: They are physiologically fundamentally different. They don't use oxygen in their muscles, dissipate heat, or raise their heart rate the same way adults do. This means that a lot of what we might do for ourselves, such as weight training or long-distance running, is not appropriate for children. It won't help them build muscle or improve performance.

One thing many adults and children do have in common when it comes to exercise is that they don't drink enough to stay well hydrated. Not hydrating well, or not getting enough sodium, can cause muscle ache in the very athletic child—especially a child who participates in activities like soccer or tennis tournaments, where multiple games are played in a day. Your child should be able to urinate before he goes to that second game. This is one way you can tell if he is hydrated enough.

Teach your child to drink *before* she gets thirsty. To keep sodium levels up, offer half water, half sports drink. If your child doesn't like sports drinks, she could drink water and eat salty foods such as pretzels or popcorn in between games. Also teach your child to warm up to begin forming good habits for later in life. Teach her to start slow, warm up, and then stretch a bit before exercise, then stretch again after the activity. This becomes more important as kids get older and will be an essential habit for them to have by adulthood.

WHEN TO CALL THE DOCTOR

Call your doctor if your child's pain is accompanied by enough swelling to limit motion; fever; rash; or other symptoms that might suggest something beyond growing pains or a simple sports injury. Also call if the pain won't go away or is getting worse rather than better despite your efforts to treat it.

If your child's pain is constant—particularly at night—or if it lasts more than four to six weeks, seek medical attention, as kids don't normally experience this type of chronic pain.

Nausea and Stomachache

Stomachaches are probably the most common childhood complaint," says Gregory T. Penny, M.D., of Boys Town National Research Hospital. Luckily, most are short-lived, lasting under an hour and requiring no medical treatment whatsoever. They can be caused by anything from nervousness or constipation to too much time running around in the sun.

Nausea, another common stomach complaint, is a symptom of many different types of illness. However, if the illness is anything beyond a common stomach virus—which generally lasts from twenty-four to forty-eight hours and resolves itself on its own—there will be other symptoms. Overheating, overactivity, motion sickness, and foods that upset the stomach can also cause nausea and vomiting; these causes don't require medical treatment, either.

Motion Sickness

If your child complains of nausea in the car and isn't otherwise ill, it is most likely due to motion sickness. This most commonly affects kids ages three to twelve, though doctors say that almost anyone can get motion sickness under the right circumstances.

Symptoms include abdominal discomfort, dizziness, tiredness, nausea, sweating, increased secretions in the mouth, flushed skin, and vomiting. Anxiety and fear, underlying poor health, bad ventilation in the vehicle or strong odors, and some medications, such as antibiotics that tend to cause nausea, can all contribute to the problem. When the motion is removed, your child should get better. However, symptoms can last as long as a day after the motion stops.

Try not to have a big meal before you go traveling. Small meals with low-fat foods are better than a greasy hamburger and french fries. Snacking on pretzels or other salty foods will dry the mouth and reduce nausea. Hard lemon candy can also help.

—MERIDITH SONNETT, M.D.,
CHILDREN'S HOSPITAL OF NEW YORK

To help keep your child from getting sick, make sure she has fresh air. If you're in the car, open a window. On boats, stay on the top deck. In airplanes, aim the vent to blow on her. If your child is old enough, sitting in the front seat of the car will help. Or put your child in the middle of the backseat, where she can see ahead, rather than looking out the side windows. Don't let your child sit in seats that face backward on cars, trains, or buses. The middle of a boat is best; on an airplane, seats over the wing tend to be most stable. Try to keep your child as still as possible, and don't do anything where you have to focus, such as playing car games or reading.

(continued)

Have your child keep the horizon in view by looking into a distant field to count cows or something else far afield. Closing her eyes and lying down might also help.

—CARLA GIANNONI, M.D.,
UNIVERSITY OF FLORIDA COLLEGE OF MEDICINE

Giving Coca-Cola, ginger ale, or candied ginger can help, because both Coke syrup and ginger are antiemetics. Many pediatricians also recommend over-the-counter medications for motion sickness. You can use antihistamines if they make your child sleepy, or Dramamine if your child is older than two. There are also prescription medications that can help.

The trick is to treat early, because once your child actually gets sick, it's harder to stop it.

—MERIDITH SONNETT, M.D.,
CHILDREN'S HOSPITAL OF NEW YORK

You might also try having your child wear acupressure wrist bands. These elastic bands, available over the counter in many pharmacies and travel stores, have disks that press against the acupressure points that relieve nausea. They are painless and work quite well for some people, according to Denise Salerno, M.D., F.A.A.P., of Temple University Children's Medical Center in Philadelphia, Pennsylvania. And if you know that your child gets sick after an hour in the car, try stopping around forty-five minutes into the trip for a leisurely break as a preventative measure.

Keep your car in good condition. If you have bad shocks, there is more sensation of up-and-down motion, which is much more problematic for kids with motion sickness than straightforward motion.

—DENISE SALERNO, M.D., F.A.A.P.,
TEMPLE UNIVERSITY CHILDREN'S MEDICAL CENTER,
PHILADELPHIA, PENNSYLVANIA

If you know your child is prone to motion sickness and vomiting, you should also be prepared with something to catch the mess. If your child vomits in the car, riding with the smell for the rest of the trip may make everyone else nauseous, too.

An air-sick bag like they have on airplanes is ideal if you think your child will be sick in the car, but avoid plastic bags because of the danger of suffocation if the child puts the bag over his head. You could also carry a large plastic bowl with a lid, so that you can put the lid on and contain the mess and smell until you can empty the bowl.

—DENISE SALERNO, M.D., F.A.A.P.,
TEMPLE UNIVERSITY CHILDREN'S MEDICAL
CENTER, PHILADELPHIA, PENNSYLVANIA

If your child's motion sickness doesn't get better when the motion stops, seek medical attention to be sure there isn't some other illness at work. If the motion sickness is so severe that it impacts your child's daily life (he can't get on the bus to go to school, or go anywhere in the car), talk to your pediatrician.

Serious causes of stomach pain and upset, including appendicitis and bowel obstruction, will need treatment, but these are much more rare, according to doctors.

FIRST RESPONSE

DO NOTHING

Believe it or not, doctors say that the most common mistake parents make if their child complains of a stomachache or nausea is to rush to try to "do something." If your child complains of stomach pain or nausea, first bring her into a comfortable environment and make sure she isn't overheated from running around too much.

> Don't make a big deal of minor symptoms, or you'll find that your child frequently complains of minor symptoms.
> —GREGORY T. PENNY, M.D.,
> BOYS TOWN NATIONAL RESEARCH HOSPITAL,
> OMAHA, NEBRASKA

Find out if your child has fever, vomiting, or diarrhea, especially if you know that there is a viral illness going around. Check to see whether your child needs to go to the bathroom, because constipation (see "Constipation") is a big cause of stomach pain in young children. "I wish I had a dollar for every time parents rushed to the hospital for a child's stomach pains, and the kid had a big poop in the ER. It's embarrassing for everybody, and it costs them five hundred dollars," says Jeffrey Penso, M.D., F.A.A.P., of Mattel Children's Hospital at UCLA.

If your child isn't constipated, comfort and reassure him and have him lie down and rest for twenty to thirty minutes. Children, especially young ones, often complain of stomach pain if they are bored or somehow uncomfortable. If your child is anxious to get up before the time is over, you know his complaint wasn't serious. However, if his pain is enough to interfere with his regular activity, it merits attention.

COMFORT CARE

If your child shows signs of dehydration—dry eyes and mouth, or decreased urine output—or has severe abdominal pain, call your doctor. Otherwise you can wait twenty-four to thirty-six hours to see if her condition improves. Simple changes in diet can help make your child more comfortable if she's vomiting.

MEDICATIONS

In general, doctors don't recommend over-the-counter medications for nausea and stomach pain. Many, they say, are not effective and are usually not necessary. If your child has a stomach virus, the only thing that will actually clear it up is "tincture of time." In other words, you have to wait for it to take its course. If your child has something more serious, such as appendicitis, over-the-counter medications will only cover up the symptom and delay your inevitable trip to the doctor.

In cases of stomach pain, doctors particularly warn against pain relievers containing ibuprofen and acetaminophen, as they are known to cause stomach upset and can actually make the problem worse. Some doctors say that Pepto-Bismol is safe and effective, though others advise avoiding it because it contains aspirin. Giving aspirin-containing products to a child with a virus can increase the danger of Reye's syndrome, a potentially fatal complication.

If your child has nausea, antacids can sometimes help but also might mask signs of a more serious condition. Don't give them unless your child's symptoms are fairly minor, and don't use them long-term. Also avoid antinausea medications, which are rarely effective in children and can mask other symptoms. Besides, doctors say that kids often feel better after they just go ahead and vomit.

If you have an infant who has gas pain or spits up after he eats, there are plenty of over-the-counter medicines that claim they can solve your problem. Most of them don't do a lot, but doctors say they are generally safe. About half of infants spit up a lot, which isn't a problem if they are otherwise generally healthy.

FLUIDS AND FOODS

If your child is vomiting—especially if he also has diarrhea (see "Diarrhea") and/or fever (see "Fever")—be careful to give enough fluids to keep him from getting dehydrated. However, don't try to do this too soon: Rushing to pour fluids down the throat of a child who has just vomited is only likely to make him vomit again. Instead, do nothing for the first half hour. Then, if your child's vomiting has stopped at least temporarily, you can start to give small amounts of clear fluids.

If your child is having a lot of vomiting, two or three hours with nothing in the stomach is fine. Then start by offering half an ounce to an ounce of fluid every fifteen minutes, and gradually increase this. Children who have been vomiting are often very thirsty. If you give them a glass with twelve ounces in it, they will drink it all down and then vomit it back up.

—GREGORY T. PENNY, M.D.,
BOYS TOWN NATIONAL RESEARCH HOSPITAL,
OMAHA, NEBRASKA

If your child has severe vomiting or vomiting with diarrhea and fever, give an electrolyte solution to keep her hydrated. You can mix this with small amounts of 7UP or another flavoring if your child doesn't like it, but it's better to use it straight if you can because the electrolyte solution has the right mix of sodium and electrolytes. You might have better luck with frozen pops made from electrolyte solutions, which you can buy or make yourself. It is important to maintain the proper sodium and electrolyte balance in the body. Giving only plain water if your child is losing a lot of fluids can lead to an imbalance serious enough to cause seizures.

Once your child can tolerate clear fluids, you can start slowly introducing the BRAT diet, a time-tested regimen of bananas, rice, applesauce, and toast. Avoid giving fruit juices, which have high levels of sugar that can cause diarrhea. It's also a good idea to avoid dairy products, which are more difficult to digest. Instead, try offering bland, starchy solid foods such as bread, grains, rice, yogurt, and pasta. Once your child can tolerate the BRAT diet, you can gradually return him to a normal diet.

WHEN TO CALL THE DOCTOR

If your child is complaining of severe pain, or isn't starting to improve after half an hour of rest and small sips of clear fluid, call your doctor. In this case, you have to consider the possibility of complications like appendicitis.

Also call the doctor if your child appears dehydrated. The signs include crying without tears, not urinating as much as normal, dry mouth and eyes, and in serious cases a sunken or hollow appearance to the face.

If your child has chronic problems with vomiting or heartburn, experiences neck pain along with nausea, vomits blood, or has blood in her stool, she might have a condition called gastroesophageal reflux. This causes stomach acid to back up into the esophagus and requires medical treatment.

Gastroesophageal Reflux

According to the Pediatric/Adolescent Gastroesophageal Reflux Association (PAGER), a nonprofit organization that provides information and support to parents, patients, and doctors, the following are the signs of GER:

- Pain, irritability, constant or sudden crying, colic
- Frequent spitting up or vomiting
- Vomiting or spitting up more than one hour after eating
- Not outgrowing the spitting-up stage
- Poor sleep habits, frequent waking
- "Wet burp" or "wet hiccup" sounds

You can contact PAGER for further information through their main office at (301) 601-9541; their West Coast office at (760) 747-5001; or their website at www.reflux.org.

Sinusitis

If your child has a runny nose from a cold or allergies and seems to be getting worse rather than better, she may have sinusitis. This is a bacterial infection of the sinuses—air pockets that are located above, below, and behind the eyes and are connected to the nasal passages. Swelling from allergies or an upper respiratory infection blocks the opening between the nasal passages and the sinus and traps fluid in these pockets, which become infected.

There are approximately 30 to 40 million cases of sinusitis per year in the United States, 10 to 20 million of which are likely children, according to Robert L. Roberts, M.D., Ph.D., of Mattel Children's Hospital at UCLA. And though cases of sinusitis are common in children, they aren't as frequent as ear infections.

FIRST RESPONSE

STOPPING NOSE STUFFERS

If your child has sinusitis, he likely has allergies, or colds more often than normal. Even if your child's current case of sinusitis clears up, if you don't prevent the colds and treat the allergies, the sinusitis will probably just come back.

> Because kids who have lots of colds and runny noses have more trouble with sinusitis, you should look at the environment in your home to see if something there might be causing the problem. Look for allergies and allergens, especially in your child's room. Consider your indoor air quality. Don't smoke in the home. Make sure the heating and air-conditioning filters are of good quality and changed frequently.
>
> —DAVID CHAIT, M.D.,
> BOYS TOWN NATIONAL RESEARCH HOSPITAL,
> OMAHA, NEBRASKA

According to doctors, you can decrease your child's allergies or colds by looking at her environment. If she is in day care and catches a lot of colds, take a look at the facility's policies and the number of children in each classroom. Facilities with strict rules about cleanliness and allowing sick children or caregivers to attend, and those with the fewest number of children, will expose your child to fewer germs.

> If your child is prone to sinusitis, you might want to avoid extreme cold temperatures. These tend to cause runny nose, which can make sinusitis worse.
>
> —ROBERT L. ROBERTS, M.D., PH.D.,
> MATTEL CHILDREN'S HOSPITAL AT UCLA

If your child has allergies, treating them might prevent sinusitis from developing. Some changes in your home will also limit the number of allergens in the air and relieve some of the irritation to your child's sinuses.

COMFORT CARE

Sinusitis is treated with a course of antibiotics, generally the same ones used to treat middle-ear infection. Sometimes the course of antibiotics runs as long as six weeks. Only occasionally will a child have a blockage or immunodeficiency that is causing a chronic problem and requires more extensive treatment.

SPOTTING THE SYMPTOMS

Sinusitis in kids can be difficult to diagnose, even for medical professionals with a sinus X ray. That's because colds and allergies cause some fluid to be trapped in the sinuses, but without taking a specimen of that fluid, it's impossible to tell whether it is infected with bacteria.

In addition, children with sinusitis often have different symptoms than adults; they aren't as likely to get the same facial pain, pressure, and headache. Rarely, kids with sinusitis will complain of a headache, especially a point headache where it hurts directly behind or around the eyes or forehead, but it is not all that common.

Kids are more likely to have a chronic cough, sore throat, and bad breath, which is caused by the bacteria draining down the back of the throat. The cough is often worse at night or when the child is lying down. They also might have fever, lethargy, or irritability and are generally sicker than kids who have a cold or allergies.

Parents often mistakenly think their child has sinusitis based on the color of the nasal secretions, but this isn't a very reliable way to tell. Doctors say there are actually two aspects to determining whether your child has sinusitis. The first is the severity of the symptoms: If your child has cold symptoms that are out of proportion to his usual illness, you might suspect sinusitis. Second is the duration of the illness: A cold that lasts longer than ten days with no improvement may be sinusitis.

Some parents tend to think that all runny noses are sinusitis, but most are not. Especially under age three, lots of kids have chronic runny noses, and this condition is not often sinusitis. It can be caused by allergies, environmental factors such as smoking in the home, or dry heat.

CLEARING THE CONGESTION

Since congestion is the main reason behind both the sinusitis infection and its ensuing discomfort, clearing it up can help prevent cases and make your child feel better if he has it. This means hydrating your child to thin nasal secretions as much as possible, and keeping the nasal passages clear. (See "Congestion and Runny Nose.")

> Steam can help relieve congestion and discomfort— especially in the morning. Try putting your child in the bathroom with a hot shower running.
>
> —JOSEPH HADDAD, JR., M.D.,
> CHILDREN'S HOSPITAL OF NEW YORK

Doctors recommend using a humidifier if your home has heating or air-conditioning that dries out the air, or if you live in an especially dry climate. You can also allow your child to sleep in a more upright position so that the mucus drains down, rather than pooling in the nasal passages and causing stuffiness.

When teaching your children to blow their noses, get
them to imagine blowing a candle out with the nose.
It's easiest for them to learn and practice while they are
healthy.
—RODNEY P. LUSK, M.D.,
ST. LOUIS CHILDREN'S HOSPITAL

If you have a very young child, you might want to suction his nose to help keep it clear. When suctioning, put
some saline in first. If the child really resists, however, doctors
say you might as well give up. Kids really have to cooperate
for suctioning to be effective. With older kids, you can use
saline nose spray to loosen congestion, then have them gently
blow their nose.

Decongestants

Don't use nasal sprays for a prolonged period of time
because of the danger of the rebound effect. And avoid
antihistamines, which can make the problem worse by
thickening the secretions.
—RODNEY P. LUSK, M.D.,
ST. LOUIS CHILDREN'S HOSPITAL

When using nasal decongestant sprays, use a pump
sprayer rather than drops. Have your child wash down
the bad taste with whatever she likes to drink. There's
no need to restrict milk if your child has sinusitis. Some
people think it will make the secretions thicker, but this
is a myth. Kids need to be as well hydrated as possible
to keep nasal secretions thin, so give them whatever
they want to drink.
—HARVEY KAGAN, M.D.,
CHILDREN'S HOSPITAL OF THE KING'S DAUGHTERS,
NORFOLK, VIRGINIA

If your child has sinusitis and allergies, many doctors like to treat them with nasal steroid sprays, which are available by prescription and reduce inflammation without thickening nasal secretions the way antihistamines can.

When using a nasal spray, aim up and toward the outer corner of the eye rather than just straight up, so that you're directing the spray toward the sinus passages. If your child finds the nasal spray uncomfortable, you can try switching brands. It's usually the preservatives rather than the active ingredient that tends to cause a burning sensation, so finding one with a different preservative might help. Ask your pharmacist.

—JOSEPH HADDAD, JR., M.D.,
CHILDREN'S HOSPITAL OF NEW YORK

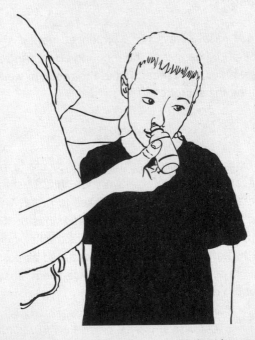

Proper way to aim a nasal spray toward the sinus passages.

Headache

Using saline drops, humidifiers, or a topical nasal decongestant to help relieve nasal congestion and pressure will often
go a long way toward relieving any pain your child might
feel. Over-the-counter analgesics can also help.

> If your child has pain from sinusitis, sitting up is more
> comfortable than lying down. Steam and hot packs are
> helpful, as is sitting in a warm bath or shower. Tylenol
> can help, and nasal decongestants can help relieve the
> pressure.
>
> —DAVID CHAIT, M.D.,
>   BOYS TOWN NATIONAL RESEARCH HOSPITAL,
>   OMAHA, NEBRASKA

Over-the-counter pain relievers can also help reduce the
fever that often accompanies sinusitis, which will make your
child feel generally better. You can give acetaminophen or
ibuprofen to help relieve the pain, just read the packaging and
keep careful track of how much you give and when. Overdoses
of these medications can be serious. Sudafed might also be
helpful, because it is a decongestant and can help relieve pressure. Drinking warm liquids can make kids feel better as well.

WHEN TO CALL THE DOCTOR

Call your child's doctor if you suspect sinusitis, because it isn't
likely to clear up without antibiotic treatment. However,
don't go in expecting to walk out with a prescription, because
only one in every six or seven colds on average turns out to be
sinusitis. Signs of possible sinus infection include:

- A cold lasting longer than ten days
- A cold or allergy symptoms with a high fever

- A cold or allergy symptoms that are getting worse
- Swelling around the eyes

Cases of acute sinusitis generally last from three to four weeks. However, sinusitis can be recurrent, and cases can overlap. Continued infection after three months is considered chronic. In this event, doctors often prescribe broader-spectrum antibiotics for a longer period of time. They also often use steroid nasal sprays to help with congestion.

> If your child has asthma (see "Asthma"), you should probably call sooner rather than later. Sinusitis can aggravate your child's asthma.
> —ROBERT L. ROBERTS, M.D., PH.D.,
> MATTEL CHILDREN'S HOSPITAL AT UCLA

If a child has chronic sinusitis, the doctor might consider removing the adenoids—small glands like tonsils, located at the back of the nose. This is a short, outpatient procedure not generally associated with pain or bleeding.

However, doctors say that you don't necessarily have to go after very aggressive treatment if your child gets lots of colds that don't make him very ill. Consider looking into other factors, such as allergies or indoor air quality, and keep in mind that many kids start to see a huge reduction in sinus problems by age four because their immune system is better developed and the openings into the sinus are larger.

Sleep Problems

One of the first questions people ask new parents is "Is the baby sleeping through the night?" That's because the state that dreams are made in is essential both for parents and their children. Though sleep requirements vary by age and individual, the consequences of not getting enough are clear. In people of all ages, lack of sleep can lead to increased stress and decreased ability to fight infection. Memory storage is entirely dependent on sleep, which means that if you don't sleep at night, your brain fails to store information it gathered during the day into the long-term memory. In babies and children under age seven, sleep is also important for proper physical growth and brain development.

In children specifically, doctors say that sleep restriction impacts behavior, cognitive abilities, and motor abilities. Unlike adults who become sleepy and lethargic, overtired children practically fight to keep themselves awake. This means they become hyperactive and "wired," fidget and misbehave, and are basically just no fun to be around. As sleep restriction increases, a child's ability to concentrate and remember things decreases, sometimes even leading to poor performance in school. Sleep-deprived children are also sloppy and accident-prone, often falling or spilling and bumping into things.

Because sleep is the body's and brain's time to rest and reorganize, your child must get a good night's sleep on a regular basis. And a child who is sleep-deprived needs more than one night to "catch up."

FIRST RESPONSE

SLEEPING LIKE A BABY

According to most doctors, the key to dealing with sleep problems is establishing good sleep habits in the first place. "As parents, we want our children to go to bed without resistance, and we want them to sleep through the night," says Matilda Garcia, M.D., of St. Joseph's Hospital in Phoenix. "But good sleep habits will not develop unless the parent has a plan." The process begins, doctors say, as soon as you bring your baby home from the hospital.

> The most important thing is to put babies down to fall asleep on their own. This is a learned habit and won't come naturally. Start at two weeks of age, and put them in bed while their eyes are still open. You can rock or hold them until they get drowsy, but not until they fall asleep.
> —SHARON BEAL, M.D.,
> MEDICAL COLLEGE OF GEORGIA

First, there's the matter of what you do when you put your baby down to sleep. Many parents are inclined to feed, rock, sing, or walk until those little eyes close, and then sneak the baby into the crib. However, most doctors advise against these activities. People of all ages have times when they wake at night and need to put themselves back to sleep. A baby who doesn't learn how to do this often ends up as an adult who is wakeful and sleeps poorly, or who can't get back to sleep once he is awake. Be aware that it takes newborns about twenty minutes of restlessness before they'll settle down and go to sleep, but instilling the good habit is worth the wait.

> Babies come home from the hospital with no sense of night and day. To help them develop one, and to help them learn to sleep through some noise, don't have their room as dark and quiet during daytime naps as you would at night. If the baby is napping, your life needs to go on. Don't turn off the phone or send your other children out of the house.
>
> —GINA DIRENZO-COFFEY, M.D.,
> BOYS TOWN NATIONAL RESEARCH HOSPITAL,
> OMAHA, NEBRASKA

Also important is the way parents treat nap time. For babies, naps are an important part of the sleep schedule, and doctors stress that keeping your baby up all day will *not* guarantee that she will sleep through the night. Just like any overtired child, a baby who hasn't had enough sleep will become wound up and unable to settle down and rest. Doctors do recommend that parents set some reasonable limits on the length of a baby's nap, and not encourage too much daytime sleep.

At night, parents should do all they can to help the baby learn that it's time for sleeping. Doctors recommend that you keep middle-of-the-night contact "brief and boring," so the baby doesn't get the idea that Mom and Dad are there to play.

Turn on as little light as possible to help you see to change the diaper or feed or check on the baby. Do what needs doing and head back to bed.

> Don't let your baby nap for more than three continuous hours during the day, and try to carry or hold her for at least three hours a day while she is *not* crying. Studies show this creates a more satisfied baby who will be less reluctant to go to sleep.
> —MATILDA GARCIA, M.D.,
> ST. JOSEPH'S HOSPITAL AND MEDICAL CENTER,
> PHOENIX

> At around six months of age, a child starts to develop patterns for eating, playing, toileting, etc. Work his sleep habits into this pattern and make it as predictable as possible. Encourage routine throughout the day, because if the rest of the day is irregular, his sleep is going to be irregular, too.
> —ZEENAT Q. MALIK, M.D.,
> ST. JOSEPH'S CHILDREN'S HOSPITAL, NEW JERSEY

Unless your baby is having problems with diaper rash (see "Diaper Rash"), or is extremely wet or uncomfortable, there is no need to routinely change his diapers in the middle of the night.

The idea is for all of this to become part of a regular sleep routine for the whole family. If you put older children to bed at the same time every night, keep your baby up late enough to have his last feeding at your bedtime, and go to bed at the same time every night yourself, you will promote good sleep habits for everyone. Then, if there are problems later on, you'll at least have a good "normal" routine as a baseline.

COMFORT CARE

Everyone has trouble sleeping sometimes—and when children don't sleep, neither do their parents. However, if you provide the proper environment and good sleep hygiene, and are consistent in how you handle sleep problems, you'll have an easier time navigating the rough patches.

THE SLEEP SPOT

There are three words to keep in mind regarding the spot where your child sleeps: safe, dark (or mostly dark), and quiet. For babies, "safe" means putting your child to sleep on his back in a crib with a firm mattress, no lead paint, and government-approved slats that are close enough together that the baby cannot slip out. For older children—especially those in bunk beds—make certain the bed is sturdy, and consider guardrails for preschoolers. If you're uncertain whether something is safe, it probably isn't.

> Kids are not going to sleep very well if they're sleeping in a different place every night. Children need a regular place to sleep.
>
> —MARY McCORD, M.D.,
> COLUMBIA PRESBYTERIAN MEDICAL CENTER

Doctors tend to agree that a child's room should be dark at night, though some say a small night-light is fine if the child needs it to feel safe. If your child is afraid of the dark, or goes through a fearful period because of nightmares, there is no harm in leaving even a larger light on for a short period of time. Wean your child away from this gradually, by leaving a smaller and smaller light on each night over a period of a week or two.

> Children should sleep in their own room instead of with
> their parents. A lot of adults snore and make noise that
> might disrupt a child's sleep. Try to reserve the bed just
> for sleep. Don't use it for punishment, time-out, or any-
> thing else.
>
> —SHARON BEAL, M.D.,
> MEDICAL COLLEGE OF GEORGIA

Your ultimate goal is to create a low-stimulus environment. The room should be quiet, nothing in it should coax
your child to get up and play. This means no exciting toys in
the child's bed and absolutely no television. Some doctors say
that soft music is fine if your child finds it soothing. Keep
older siblings with later bedtimes out of the room, as their
activity is likely to disrupt the younger child's sleep.

> Consistency is the key to a good bedtime routine. No
> wrestling, tickling, or scary stories.
>
> —ZEENAT Q. MALIK, M.D.,
> ST. JOSEPH'S CHILDREN'S HOSPITAL, NEW JERSEY

Pacifiers and Thumbs

Many babies and young children soothe themselves to sleep
by sucking on a pacifier, finger, or thumb. Both the American
Academy of Pediatrics and the American Academy of Pediatric Dentistry say this practice is completely harmless and
perfectly normal. The sucking reflex is present in all babies,
and many begin to suck on their fingers or thumbs before
they are even born.

   Your child's sucking habit is really cause for concern only
if it begins to change the shape of your child's mouth or

teeth, or persists beyond the age of six to eight years when it might impact your child's permanent teeth. Watch for changes in the roof of your child's mouth, and in the way the teeth are lining up, and talk with your doctor or pediatric dentist if you notice a problem. Regular checkups with a pediatric dentist can help detect problems early, when they are most easily corrected.

Despite concern from many parents and caregivers that giving a pacifier to a baby is harmful, the American Academy of Pediatrics maintains that it does not cause any medical or psychosocial problems. The academy does caution, however, that a pacifier should not be used to replace or delay a baby's meals.

According to the American Academy of Dentistry, thumb, finger, and pacifier sucking—including special "orthodontic" versions—all impact the teeth essentially the same way. A pacifier habit, however, might be easier to break since you can take the pacifier away from the child. Fingers and thumbs are always there.

One disadvantage to pacifier use at night is that many babies will wake up when the pacifier falls out of their mouths. Until the baby is old enough to find the pacifier on her own, someone else must get up in the middle of the night to do it. The AAP warns against tying pacifiers to your baby's crib, or around her neck or hand, because the baby could strangle in the string.

If you choose to give your child a pacifier, the AAP recommends buying a dishwasher-safe, one-piece model, with a shield that is at least 1¼ inches across. The shield should be made of firm plastic and have airholes to prevent choking. You should never use the nipple from a baby bottle as a pacifier, since the nipple could come loose from the ring and choke the baby. You should also inspect your child's pacifier every few weeks to make sure the rubber is not beginning to deteriorate. If it is, buy a new one.

TUCK-IN TIME

Sleep hygiene (a good bedtime routine) is essential in making sure your child knows when it's time to go to sleep. Doctors say that you can start to create a bedtime routine for your child as early as age one. And the more you maintain the routine, the more likely your child will be to adjust to it.

> The most important thing is to have some sort of routine that lasts fifteen to forty-five minutes before bed. Some experts recommend having your toddler say good night to all her favorite objects in the house, but any quiet activity is fine. You want your child to have a kind of Pavlovian response to whatever your routine is.
>
> —MARY McCORD, M.D.,
> COLUMBIA PRESBYTERIAN MEDICAL CENTER

Pre-bedtime needs vary from child to child. While some kids can just run in from playing, brush their teeth, put on their pajamas, and fall asleep, others need more of a transition. The best way to provide this is to schedule a set of quiet activities before bed.

> Sometimes kids who used to have good sleep habits will give them up for one reason or another (teething, travel, and illness always disrupt sleep habits). You might have to be firm with your child and even let him cry, but you're doing it for a good reason. Kids need good sleep. If your spouse objects, let him get up with your child at night from then on. This will usually get him on your side.
>
> —SHARON BEAL, M.D.,
> MEDICAL COLLEGE OF GEORGIA

Traditional bedtime activities include nursing or a bottle for babies (though you don't want your baby to fall asleep while eating because of the risks of choking and dental decay), a bath, and quiet reading. Try to do these things in the same order every night; some doctors even recommend using the same words and saying the same things ("Time to give Daddy a hug" or "Into the tub now") night after night. This establishes a comforting routine.

> For kids who really need a big transition before bed, you might even try beginning the process of quieting down their activity as early as after dinner. Do whatever matches your child.
>
> —GINA DiRENZO-COFFEY, M.D.,
> BOYS TOWN NATIONAL RESEARCH HOSPITAL,
> OMAHA, NEBRASKA

The routine doesn't have to be rigid, but it must be predictable. This way, protests will come soon—during the bath, for instance—and you can deal with them early rather than as you are putting the child into bed.

> Set limits to your child's bedtime routine, such as how many stories will be read or how many quiet activities you will do.
>
> —ZEENAT Q. MALIK, M.D.,
> ST. JOSEPH'S CHILDREN'S HOSPITAL, NEW JERSEY

Older kids need a quiet pre-bed routine, too. For instance, most kids can't go from the stimulation of playing a video game to sleeping without transition. As your child grows older, the routine will probably be more under her control, but it still might include things like a bath or shower and reading.

Make sure your routine fits well with the lifestyle of your household. If you're trying to put your child into bed at nine P.M., and that's when Dad comes home, that's not going to work. You'll need to put your child in bed either earlier or later.

—MARY McCORD, M.D.,
COLUMBIA PRESBYTERIAN MEDICAL CENTER

Obstructive Sleep Apnea

If your child is tired during the day despite the fact that he appeared to sleep all night, and if he snores heavily, obstructive sleep apnea could be the culprit. This condition makes it appear as if your child has been sleeping through the night. In reality, however, he has been waking several times a night because he snores so deeply that he ends up holding his breath for several seconds and must wake to breathe deeply. He moves around, reopens the airway, and gasps for breath. The recurrent low oxygen can cause health problems, and it doesn't let him get a good night's sleep. Some kids who suffer from this condition don't rest well, and wake up with a morning headache or don't feel good. Sleep apnea can also cause hyperactivity, inattentiveness, aggressive behavior, irritability, and mood swings, according to the American Sleep Apnea Association.

One of the main causes of apnea is enlarged adenoids. These are small glands similar to tonsils, located in the upper throat at the back of the nasal passages. When the adenoids are removed through a simple outpatient surgery, the apnea usually stops. For further information about evaluation and treatment of sleep apnea, you can visit the American Sleep Apnea Association website at www.sleepapnea.org.

COMMON SLEEP PROBLEMS

Caffeine and Sugar

If your child is having problems sleeping, avoid products containing caffeine—including chocolate, soda, and tea—after lunchtime. Avoiding them after dinner is too late, because they can impact sleep even if ingested hours before bedtime.

A big meal right before bed can also make sleeping hard, as can too much sugar in some kids. Every body is different, so be alert and try to make a note of what things interfere with your child's sleep.

> Be careful of how much your toddler drinks before bedtime. Many drink a lot and wake up because their diapers are soaking wet. Then, in order to settle them back down, the parent gives them more to drink. This can create a vicious cycle.
>
> —SHARON BEAL, M.D.,
> MEDICAL COLLEGE OF GEORGIA

Decongestants can also disrupt sleep. If congestion is a problem for your child and you must give a decongestant before bed, look for one that is packaged in combination with antihistamines, so that the sleep-inducing effect of the antihistamine balances the stimulating effect of the decongestant. Be aware, however, that some children react the opposite way to antihistamines (doctors call this a "paradoxical effect") and will actually get hyper. Test any medication you plan to give at bedtime at some earlier point during the day to judge the effect it will have on your child.

If you do find a medication that sedates your child (Benadryl, an antihistamine, is a common one), doctors warn against using it as a crutch to make your child sleep. Your child could become dependent on it and be unable to sleep without a dose.

Separation Anxiety

If your child is waking during the night between the ages of about nine and twelve months, this problem is likely caused by separation anxiety. This means she is worried about being away from you and the rest of the family while she is falling asleep; it is a fairly common problem.

> If your child has separation anxiety, try doing the separation in stages. At first, stay in the room while your child falls asleep. Next, be outside the room, but leave your child's door open. Finally, you can move to closing the bedroom door and having your child fall asleep without you.
>
> —DAVID GOZAL, M.D.,
>   KOSAIR CHILDREN'S HOSPITAL,
>   LOUISVILLE, KENTUCKY

Doctors say that separation anxiety is a normal developmental stage. It isn't your child's fault, and it isn't something to scold about. You have to try to understand what the child is going through. The tough part is that you also have to do your best to follow the bedtime routine and be consistent and firm.

Most doctors recommend a "tough love" approach. If your child cries or screams, try not to rush right into the room. Wait five minutes or so (look at your watch or set a timer). Comfort your child with calm words and a pat or rub on the back, but *do not pick him up*. Be firm, and then leave again. Be consistent with this, and do it in about ten-minute blocks. No one wants to hear a child cry, so use your watch or timer as a guide. This approach isn't for everyone, and it won't work unless both parents have agreed to do it and stick with it. Consistency is key here; if you break down after a few minutes and pick up your child, you're actually training her to keep crying no matter what, since she'll learn that you'll come in eventually.

Some doctors also suggest a transitional object to help younger kids deal with a sleep problem. Having that special toy or stuffed animal, perhaps one offered only at bedtime, makes bedtime positive. They're happy to see the toy and know that it signifies bedtime. Whatever you try, be consistent in your approach. Trying different things night after night will only confuse your child and could increase his anxiety about bedtime.

Sleepwalking

Sleepwalking of some sort affects at least 20 to 30 percent of children at one point or another, according to doctors. It usually starts around age three to four and is outgrown by age eight or nine. It doesn't suggest anything wrong with your child, and there isn't much you can do to prevent it.

Instead, make sure your child is safe. This means putting gates on stairs, keeping floors and hallways clear of tripping hazards, and putting away potentially dangerous objects. However, don't lock your child's bedroom door. This is dangerous because it could interfere with the child reaching you in an emergency.

Hang a bell on your child's bedroom door, so that if she leaves the room, you can hear her. If you find her sleepwalking and she's agitated, don't try to restrain her unless she's approaching something dangerous. This could make her more agitated, and you or your child might be hurt. Instead, just wait until she calms down, and then gently guide her back to bed.

—ZEENAT Q. MALIK, M.D.,
ST. JOSEPH'S CHILDREN'S HOSPITAL, NEW JERSEY

Once you return your child to bed, she'll probably settle down and keep right on sleeping. Don't be alarmed if she doesn't recognize you (remember, she's sleeping), and don't try to wake her. It is a myth that waking a sleepwalker is dangerous, but doing so could agitate and confuse your child.

Nightmares and Night Terrors

Nightmares and night terrors might both cause your child to wake you with a scream, but they are completely different things. Nightmares are bad dreams that make your child wake up and feel afraid. Night terrors are similar to sleepwalking, in that they happen when your child is in a deep sleep. They won't usually wake your child.

> Night terrors tend to run in spells. Your child won't have any and will then go through a period of having them frequently. One good way to break the cycle is to put your child to bed and wake him after an hour, then let him go back to sleep. This will prevent him from going into that deepest stage of sleep that usually brings about the night terror.
>
> —SHARON BEAL, M.D.,
> MEDICAL COLLEGE OF GEORGIA

If your child happens to wake you while he's having a night terror, try to remember that the experience is likely more frightening for you than for your child. It's not like a nightmare. Your child probably won't wake or remember anything, so don't try too hard to comfort him unless he actually wakes. When your child has night terrors, remember that he won't recognize you the moment he wakes up. Keep him from hurting himself, but don't try to hold him if he doesn't want to be held. The best thing to do is wait them out.

Night terrors and sleepwalking can sometimes occur more frequently in times of stress, but doctors aren't sure exactly what causes them. Nightmares, on the other hand, can often be triggered by something your child saw in a movie or on television, or by a story she heard from a friend. We all dream four to five times a night to help our minds process complicated information, but we don't always remember our dreams, and we all have the occasional nightmare. Doctors theorize that because children spend more time than adults in the dream state, they are more likely to have nightmares. Studies show that exposure to violent media also increases the incidence of nightmares. Figuring out the cause might help the nightmares stop.

> It will be easier to convince your child that you will be there to protect him than it will be to convince him that monsters aren't real. To children, monsters are real.
>
> —ZEENAT Q. MALIK, M.D.,
> ST. JOSEPH'S CHILDREN'S HOSPITAL, NEW JERSEY

Children often have nightmares about unrealistic things, such as monsters or aliens coming to take them away. If your child wakes with a nightmare like this, many doctors warn against practices like checking under the bed or in the closet to prove to your child that nothing is there. Doing so only shows your child that you believe in monsters, and that though nothing is there now, something might show up later. Instead, comfort your child and tell him he is safe at home with you.

If your child is having a nightmare about something more realistic, such as losing a parent, reassure her that it was just a bad dream and that everything is fine. However, try to figure out the next day what triggered the dream. Recurring nightmares can be a sign of some type of emotional disturbance.

The day after a nightmare, help your child talk about the dream and have her draw a picture or write a story about the dream. Encourage her to finish it with a happy ending. I used to tell my daughter, when she was a child, to imagine that she had wings so that she could fly away from whatever was chasing her.

—MATILDA GARCIA, M.D.,
ST. JOSEPH'S HOSPITAL AND MEDICAL CENTER,
PHOENIX

If your child is having a nightmare about a particular fear, try reading a book about that fear. The book might provide help in and of itself, and also will provide an opportunity for your child to talk more about what's bothering her. At good children's bookstores, the staff should be able to provide a book about whatever fear your child might have.

—MARY McCORD, M.D.,
COLUMBIA PRESBYTERIAN MEDICAL CENTER

Children who wake up frightened by nightmares must learn to soothe themselves back to sleep. When your child wakes from a nightmare, doctors say you should calm and reassure her, but don't pick her up or move her from her bed. This will disrupt her sleep routine. If you're going to have a long discussion about the dream, leave it until morning.

The next morning, let your child tell you the story of the nightmare if he wants, talk about it, and answer any questions he might have. Do your best to figure out together what's triggering the nightmare. Sometimes helping your child see how her brain knits together frightening or confusing images from wake time into dream time will dispel the fear.

If your child doesn't want to go to bed because of a nightmare, sometimes using a transitional object—such as a stuffed animal—or offering to use a night-light or leave the bedroom door open, might help. You might also try sitting in a chair beside the bed until she falls asleep. The next night, move the chair farther away from the bed; the next, just outside the door. Continue gradually moving farther away until your child is again comfortable falling asleep on her own.

WHEN TO CALL THE DOCTOR

Your main concern if your child is having sleep problems is that both your child and the family need to get some rest. Everyone needs a regular good night's sleep in order to be healthy. However, there are some other health problems that might be connected with your child's lack of sleep.

If you hear her snoring more than two or three times per week, or if she is often sleepy during the day without an apparent reason (such as attending a sleepover the night before), your child could have obstructive sleep apnea. This is a condition where the child's breathing is somehow blocked— sometimes by enlarged adenoids—forcing her to wake several times a night to breathe. The child won't likely wake completely, so probably won't notice the condition. Doctors also report that excessive daytime sleepiness can be a preliminary sign of narcolepsy, a sleeping disorder that causes uncontrollable sleepiness and frequent daytime sleeping.

If your child is having a sleep problem, keep a sleep diary for his doctor. Gather information on when your child naps and when he wakes up at night. Note the time so that you can give accurate information. Many parents say their child was up for an hour when he was up for only fifteen minutes; it just *felt* like an hour.

—MATILDA GARCIA, M.D.,
ST. JOSEPH'S HOSPITAL AND MEDICAL CENTER,
PHOENIX

Contact your doctor if your child behaves oddly during sleep, such as crying out or moving in an unusual way. This could indicate a seizure. Videotape the behavior if it's recurring. Thirty percent of seizures manifest only during sleep.

Since your child's sleep problem doesn't have to be caused by a serious condition to cause serious trouble for your family, check with your doctor if you're having trouble establishing a comfortable sleep routine for your child, or if something happens to interrupt your child's sleep routine—such as a vacation or an illness—and you can't get back to normal in a week or two. If your child is having severe separation issues, or any other sleep problem that is becoming disruptive to the family, don't wait to get help.

The Rules of Sleep

As important as a good night's sleep is for both kids and parents, it might not seem meant to be, especially in the early years of a child's life. The conflict starts when the maternity and paternity leave is over and Mom and Dad have to return to work. "There's a conflict between society and the true physiologic needs of the parent, because the parent who is caring for a baby who wakes up to eat every three hours still has to get up in the morning and go to work," says David Gozal, M.D., of Kosair Children's Hospital. Because children's normal sleep patterns don't generally match those of their parents until around age eight, the parents lose out in the beginning.

Don't worry too much about the number of hours of sleep your child gets. The amount needed varies from person to person. As long as he isn't tired during the day, he's getting enough.

—MATILDA GARCIA, M.D.,
ST. JOSEPH'S HOSPITAL AND MEDICAL CENTER,
PHOENIX

Doctors say it's unusual to see a child who's truly sleep-deprived in the early years. One thing that might get in the way of an early-elementary-age child getting enough sleep is the school schedule. According to Gozal, even children around the age of six could sometimes use a little nap in the afternoon, but if the child's school doesn't schedule nap time, he has to stay awake.

> You need to get enough sleep, but there's not a moral imperative to doing it a certain way. If you keep your toddler up until midnight because you don't get home from work until ten P.M., that's okay as long as she gets to sleep late or gets a nap during the day. Just be aware that once your child starts school, this routine will no longer work.
>
> —MARY MCCORD, M.D.,
> COLUMBIA PRESBYTERIAN MEDICAL CENTER

As your child gets older, she is more likely to end up sleep-deprived than you. Adolescents sometimes stay up late to watch certain television shows or because they have so much homework that they must stay up to get it done. In addition, teenagers often take part-time jobs that require them to work late. If you notice behavior changes in your adolescent or teen, or if lack of sleep is impacting your child's schoolwork, consult your doctor.

Sore Throat

Throats don't get much attention—until they're sore. And then that scratchy, achy pain that makes it tough to talk and swallow can make the rest of the body feel pretty miserable, too. Most sore throats, doctors say, are in some way related to a viral infection. Nasal drainage caused by an upper respiratory infection or allergies can run down the back of the throat and cause irritation. And if a child is forced to breathe only through his mouth because his nose is so congested, the throat can become dry and irritated.

A bigger worry for parents, however, is the dreaded strep throat. But only about 10 percent of sore throats are caused by strep infections, according to Harvey Kagan, M.D., of Children's Hospital of the King's Daughters in Norfolk, Virginia. A lab test is the only way to tell for sure if a child's sore throat is from a strep infection, doctors say. Most sore throats not caused by strep infection run their course in a few days, before test results even come back.

FIRST RESPONSE

SIGNS OF STREP THROAT

Though strep throat is one of the less-common causes of sore throat, it does require antibiotic treatment. You'll want to watch for signs of strep infection so you know whether your child needs to visit the doctor, or whether you can treat her sore throat at home.

Signs of strep infection:

- mild to severe sore throat
- muffled voice
- fever of 101 degrees or higher
- headache
- abdominal pain or vomiting
- enlarged lymph glands in the neck under the jaw
- enlarged, red tonsils, sometimes with yellow or white mucus on them
- usually, no cough or runny nose

COMFORT CARE

Children tend to complain of less pain from sore throats than adults and don't often need much in the way of at-home treatment. So if your child is complaining of extreme pain from a sore throat, it's a good reason to see your doctor. Meanwhile, there are things you can do to help make your child more comfortable.

FOR SORE THROAT WITH CONGESTION

If your child has a stuffy or runny nose with sore throat, relieving those symptoms will often help with the throat pain as well. Doctors recommend that you increase your child's fluid intake to keep the throat moist and to thin nasal secretions and make them less irritating. Increasing the humidity in your child's room with a cool-mist vaporizer will also help. Just remember to clean the machine every three days to prevent the growth and spread of mold and bacteria.

> Mix a 50-50 solution of orange juice and 7Up and give it to your child to sip. The combination of citric acid and carbonation can help clear the drainage out of the throat and provide topical relief.
> —David Chait, M.D.,
> Boys Town National Research Hospital,
> Omaha, Nebraska

You can also use an over-the-counter saline nose spray to help thin secretions and relieve congestion, or an over-the-counter decongestant to help unclog your child's nose so he doesn't have to breathe through his mouth. (See "Congestion and Stuffy Nose")

JUST PLAIN PAIN

Aside from relieving any congestion or postnasal drip that is irritating your child's throat, doctors say there is no harm in trying over-the-counter throat sprays or lozenges. You can also use that old standby, Tylenol, to help with pain.

Hard candies that have butterscotch seem to be more soothing to a sore throat than any other type.
—Harvey Kagan, M.D.,
Children's Hospital of the King's Daughters,
Norfolk, Virginia

Liquid Benadryl mixed with an equal amount of Kaopectate makes an excellent remedy for sore throat. You can give a teaspoon of this no more than four times per day, unless your child is able to gargle with the mixture and spit it out without swallowing any. A teaspoon of corn syrup can also help soothe a sore throat.
—Harvey Kagan, M.D.,
Children's Hospital of the King's Daughters,
Norfolk, Virginia

If your child is having trouble swallowing food, offer soft foods such as pudding, rice, or mashed potatoes that are less painful to get down. And make sure you serve plenty of cool liquids on the side, which doctors say are more soothing to the throat than the salt-water gargle that for years has been a home remedy for throat maladies of all sorts.

ANTIBIOTICS AND STREP TESTS

Far too many parents, according to doctors, assume that a case of sore throat means a course of antibiotics. But antibiotics won't work against the viruses that most often cause sore throat and can only help if your child has a strep infection.

Unfortunately, many parents don't know this, and take their child to the doctor practically demanding a prescription, which has led to antibiotic overuse. To determine whether antibiotics will truly help your child's sore throat, the doctor will need to perform a throat culture and strep test. This involves rubbing a soft swab against the back of the throat to gather a sample, which many kids find uncomfortable and gag-inducing.

The best approach to helping your child through a throat culture is to be direct, say doctors. Explain to them that the procedure might make them feel uncomfortable, and might make them feel like they're going to gag, but that it will be short. Tell them that the doctor will be as gentle as possible, and ask your child to try and help the doctor, so that it will be over more quickly and they can start to get better.

If the results of the strep test come back positive and you do receive a prescription for antibiotics, you must give the full course according to your doctor's instructions, and discard any leftovers. Some parents are tempted to save them for future problems, but because these medications deteriorate very fast, they aren't likely to work against another infection. In addition, if you gave the medication as prescribed, you won't have enough left over to treat another infection anyway.

WHEN TO CALL THE DOCTOR

If your child shows signs of strep throat, you'll need to make an appointment to see the doctor, who can give a strep test and prescribe antibiotics as needed. You should also call the doctor if your child—with or without signs of strep throat—has a sore throat along with the following symptoms.

- Difficulty swallowing or breathing
- Fever greater than 103 degrees Fahrenheit
- Abdominal pain
- Skin rash
- Earache

- Nasal discharge with bloody mucus
- Chest pain
- Convulsions
- Nausea or vomiting

These are all signs that something more serious than a viral infection is present. You should also call your child's doctor if the sore throat isn't accompanied by other symptoms—such as congestion, runny nose, or cough—that make its cause obvious.

Splinters

Kids naturally love to play outdoors around decks, swing sets, and wooden fences. They like to romp through the woods or garden, or build clubhouses with spare lumber. This makes them prone to get stuck with the occasional splinter.

FIRST RESPONSE

WHAT SPLINTERED

If your child comes to you with a splinter, your first concerns are where the splinter is, and how large a chunk of material you're dealing with. Large hunks of wood or metal and splinters in the face usually require medical attention and shouldn't be removed at home.

You'll also want to know where your child picked up the splinter in question. If your child was playing on a farm, near a trash dump, or someplace else that harbors a lot of dirt and germs, make sure her tetanus vaccination is up to date.

COMFORT CARE

SLIPPING OUT SPLINTERS

If your child has a smaller splinter that you plan to remove yourself, first clean the area gently with an alcohol wipe, or with soap and water if you don't have an alcohol wipe. Be careful not to press the splinter further in. There isn't anything you can do to effectively numb the area before trying to remove the splinter. If you use ice long enough to really numb the skin, you're in danger of giving your child frostbite.

Try to "milk" the splinter out by pressing your thumbs firmly on both sides of the splinter, pushing away from rather than toward the splinter. Pull the skin back, and then work gently back and forth to try to coax the splinter free. This is especially effective with splinters of glass.

—JILL S. REEL, M.D.,
BOYS TOWN NATIONAL RESEARCH HOSPITAL,
OMAHA, NEBRASKA

The ideal way to clean and sterilize your tweezers and needle is to first burn the ends in a candle flame, then clean away the soot with an alcohol wipe. If the splinter is covered over completely with a layer of skin, use a needle to try to break the skin open. Slide the needle in beside where the splinter went in, then pry up with the sharp end of the needle to cut open the skin over the splinter. Use the side of the needle to gently fold back the skin, and take the splinter out with tweezers.

How to "milk" a splinter
out of the skin.

If your child has a number of very small, superficial splinters, such as you might get from a wooden deck or swing set, you can soak the area briefly in warm water and use a washcloth to scrub them off. Bigger splinters, however, shouldn't be soaked because they can soak up water, expand, and become more difficult to remove.

—Jill S. Reel, M.D.,
Boys Town National Research Hospital,
Omaha, Nebraska

Once the splinter is out, follow up with a soap-and-water wash, antibiotic cream, and a bandage. If you think you've gotten the splinter out but your child is still complaining of pain, there could still be a piece of the splinter left under the skin. If you've tried to get a splinter out for fifteen or twenty minutes with no success, it's time to give up. That doesn't sound like a long time, but if you're in there digging and poking, it's a long time to your child. You can wait a week or two to see if the splinter works itself out, keeping the area clean with soap and water, and covering it with a bandage and antibiotic cream. However, if the skin starts to grow over the splinter, or if the area looks infected, seek medical attention.

WHEN TO CALL THE DOCTOR

Call your doctor if your child has a very large splinter—
especially in the hand or foot, or on the face—or if the splinter is so painful that your child is reluctant to use the body
part in question. When a large object is embedded in the
skin, there is a potential for nerve damage. Watch for numbness or tingling in the area.

You should also call if your child has a splinter that you
don't feel comfortable removing yourself, if a splinter isn't
working itself out within two weeks, or if your child's splinter looks infected. Signs of infection include extreme redness, pus, and worsening pain.

More frightening to look at than it is serious, a sty is a swollen red bump at the edge of the eyelid, right at the lash line. It looks like a big pimple, but a sty is really an infection of the oil glands at the base of the eyelashes. Staph or strep bacteria—with which most parents are painfully familiar because of their association with ailments like strep throat and food poisoning—are usually the cause, though the infection can also be viral.

The invading bacteria or virus causes inflammation and blockage of the gland, which then swells, reddens, and fills with pus. Sties are not highly contagious but could be spread by hand-to-eye contact. Once in a while, though not often, they are recurrent.

Sties are sometimes confused with chalazions, which are oil glands that are plugged but not infected. These are neither red nor painful and can take weeks to go away rather than days. Sometimes sties turn into chalazions before they clear up.

FIRST RESPONSE

ANTIBIOTICS OR NOT?

Doctors say that most sties can be treated at home, though it is sometimes difficult for parents to get their kids to sit still long enough and often enough for treatment to be effective. Sties can also be treated with prescription antibiotic ointments or drops, which can also be inconvenient to use but might clear up the problem more quickly.

> If there is an eyelash growing out of your child's sty, don't pull it. It's too risky and could cause infection.
> —GREGG LUEDER, M.D.,
> ST. LOUIS CHILDREN'S HOSPITAL

Doctors say that the majority of sties will take care of themselves if left alone. They will most often come to a head, burst, and drain away. However, doctors don't advise taking the risk. A sty that isn't treated could progress to an infection of the whole eyelid, for which your child will need systemic antibiotics. Or the infection might progress from an acute infection into a chronic infection where the pus changes into granulation tissue, where the tissue becomes hardened. Doctors describe that as "like having a pea under your eyelid." A chronic infection can take months to clear up.

COMFORT CARE

The pain from your child's sty will go away once the sty starts to drain. The best way to speed this along is with warm compresses—if you can get your child to sit still. You can also see your doctor for antibiotic eyedrops or ointment.

WARM SOAKS

Warm soaks are the best home treatment for sties, but they, too, aren't easy to get a small child to sit still for. They will either bring the sty to a head so that it will burst, or help it become reabsorbed into the skin.

> Create warm compresses with tap water rather than with the microwave, because heating in the microwave can cause "hot spots" [in the cloth].
> —GREGG LUEDER, M.D.,
> ST. LOUIS CHILDREN'S HOSPITAL

The compress should be as warm as your child can stand without discomfort; test it on yourself first to make sure it isn't too hot. Because five minutes is an eternity to a child, try to distract him by putting on a video or just sitting with him in front of the television and letting him watch his favorite show with the other eye. You might even try the compress in the bathtub, with tub toys as a distraction.

> If you're using a compress with warm water and a wash-cloth, it will cool off after about a minute and need to be reheated. You can put a basin of warm water nearby to reheat it, or you can use a warm boiled egg (not peeled) or baked potato wrapped in a damp washcloth instead. These stay hot longer.
> —DOUGLAS R. FREDRICK, M.D.,
> CHILDREN'S HOSPITAL AT DARTMOUTH

Doctors' recommendations for how long and how often to use the compresses range from once or twice a day, for two to five minutes, to four times a day for five to ten minutes, to "as long as you can get your child to sit still." Doctors generally concede that parents should just do the best they can. If you can manage the compress only once a day, it will still work; it just might take longer to heal the sty. You can also use a compress more often if your child lets you, which will help resolve the sty faster. If your child resists too much, some doctors say the compresses aren't worth trying at all.

> The best thing you can do to get a child to sit still for a warm compress is to offer small bribes. Even then, very few people have success. Don't feel guilty if the compresses don't work. It doesn't mean you didn't do it right. These infections tend to have a mind of their own and can drive doctors and parents crazy.
>
> —PAMELA F. GALLIN, M.D.,
> CHILDREN'S HOSPITAL OF NEW YORK

If you're successful with the warm soaks, the sty should improve within about forty-eight hours. Once the sty starts to drain, doctors recommend that you keep using compresses until it completely goes away, usually for about five days. You can give Tylenol, or another over-the-counter analgesic, to help with the pain.

ANTIBIOTIC DROPS AND OINTMENT

If warm compresses don't work on your child's sty, or you aren't comfortable trying them, you can see a pediatrician. A prescription for antibiotic eyedrops or ointment will usually clear up the sty.

Antibiotic medications are difficult to use because your child is likely to resist or to squirm while you apply them. Pamela F. Gallin, M.D., of Children's Hospital of New York, says that it's best to just apply them as quickly as possible, because the anticipation is worse than the doing. For drops, pull down the lower lid so that you can get the drop into the open eye.

> To make applying antibiotic ointment easier, hold the tube in your hand or put it in your pocket for about ten minutes before applying to warm it and make it liquefy and glide on easier. If you wash your hands, you can apply the ointment first to your finger, and then to the eye. This is easier than using a cotton swab or the applicator.
>
> —DOUGLAS R. FREDRICK, M.D.,
> CHILDREN'S HOSPITAL AT DARTMOUTH

Antibiotic (usually erythromycin) ointment can be easier to use than drops. If your child resists, goo some on the eyelashes, where it will melt and get in.

EYELID HYGIENE

Because a sty is a bacterial or viral infection, it can be contagious, so be careful to follow proper hygiene to keep it from spreading. If you've touched your child's eyes, wash your hands, and have her use separate towels from the rest of your family.

> There is no over-the-counter medication that will make a sty go away. However, if your child has a sty on the underside of the eyelid, artificial tears can help the eye feel less irritated.
>
> —DOUGLAS R. FREDRICK, M.D.,
> CHILDREN'S HOSPITAL AT DARTMOUTH

It's tough to get your child to leave a sty alone, but do the best you can. By rubbing it, he can add new bacteria to the infection or spread it to the entire eyelid. If you see your child touching or rubbing his eye, make sure he washes his hands.

If the sty comes to a head and bursts, as many do, keep the area clean with a cotton ball soaked in warm water. Talk to your doctor about using a prescription antibiotic ointment to help prevent additional infection.

> In the bathtub, first place a warm washcloth over the eye for a few minutes. Next, put a little No More Tears shampoo on the washcloth, lather, and gently wash the eyelashes.
>
> —GREGG LUEDER, M.D.,
> ST. LOUIS CHILDREN'S HOSPITAL

If your child gets recurrent sties, doctors recommend that you begin a routine of "eyelid hygiene." This involves cleaning your child's eyelashes on a regular basis, generally at night. During the day, any bacteria caught in your eyelashes gets washed away by the window-washer action of the eyelids. The secretions from your eyes rinse the lashes and help fight infection. At night, because your eyes stay closed, you don't have the window-washer effect and the bacteria can build up.

> Before your child goes to bed, mix a quarter capful of Johnson's baby shampoo and three fourths of a capful of water, and swab the eyelashes with a washcloth.
>
> —PAMELA F. GALLIN, M.D.,
> CHILDREN'S HOSPITAL OF NEW YORK

WHEN TO CALL THE DOCTOR

If your child's sty doesn't start to improve—with the red area around the base getting less red, and the sty starting to shrink—within about forty-eight hours, call your pediatrician. If you haven't tried antibiotic ointment or drops, he will likely give you a prescription. If you've been using antibiotics but they haven't helped, you might need a different antibiotic. If your child's sty lasts for as long as three months, your doctor will probably recommend a specialist to drain it. This is an outpatient procedure.

Also seek medical attention if your child has significant redness or swelling of the eyelid, if the redness spreads to other parts of the eye, if the swelling or pain is increasing, or if your child has fever, which could mean the infection has spread to the tissue around the eye. This can be serious.

If your child's whole eye is red, this could be conjunctivitis (see "Conjunctivitis"), which isn't especially serious but might require antibiotic drops. A sty or other red growth on your newborn's eye should be checked by a doctor as well.

Taking Your Child's Temperature

When a child's temperature goes up, so does a parent's blood pressure—partially because of the stress most of us associate with bringing a thermometer anywhere near our child. And while any number of new devices—from pacifiers with thermometers in the nipple to ear thermometers to thin strips of plastic held to a child's forehead—have tried to make the task easier, the fact is that doctors say the good old-fashioned way is still best. A rectal temperature with a mercury thermometer remains the gold standard when checking for fever.

COMFORT CARE

BOTTOMS UP

Most parents are as reluctant to take their child's temperature rectally as they imagine their child is to have it taken that way. But doctors stress that there's really no better way to get an

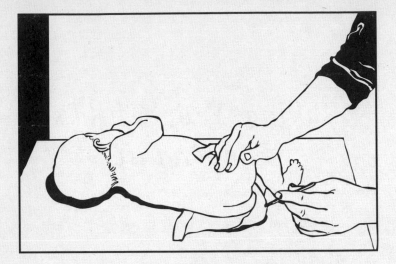

Putting baby on her side for a rectal temperature.

accurate temperature in an infant. And most say that it really isn't that difficult once you get the hang of it.

> Use K-Y Jelly to lubricate the thermometer for a rectal temperature rather than petroleum products, as these can encourage growth of bacteria. The thermometer only needs to go in about half the length of your thumb to be effective.
>
> —MATTHEW O. MCKEEVER, M.D.,
> CHILDREN'S NATIONAL MEDICAL CENTER

Use either a mercury or digital thermometer that is made for taking a rectal temperature. Don't use an oral thermometer, as they are not as sturdy and might break. If you use a mercury thermometer, make sure you shake it down below 96 degrees Fahrenheit before you begin.

There's no need to be squeamish about taking a rectal temperature. Parents need to relax. Try putting the baby on his side, bringing the knees and hips up, and just unfastening one tape of the diaper. This way, if the baby urinates during temperature taking, it won't make a mess.

—RUBY ROY, M.D.,
RONALD MCDONALD CHILDREN'S HOSPITAL
OF LOYOLA

Wash and lubricate the thermometer, and put the baby into position. Any position that is comfortable for you and your baby is fine, as long as you can keep the baby still and supported, and hold the thermometer in place.

As a mom, I found that the easiest way to take a rectal temperature was to put the baby tummy-down across my lap. That way one hand is free to support the baby, while the other holds the thermometer in place.

—ROXANNE KANE, M.D.,
CHILDREN'S HOSPITAL OF WISCONSIN

Insert the thermometer approximately half an inch, and hold it in place for the length of time recommended by the manufacturer. This is usually between two and three minutes, and some thermometers come with an automatic timer so you don't have to watch the clock.

A rectal temperature doesn't have to be that uncomfortable if you can get the child to relax. The thermometer isn't that big. Talk to your child and rub her back to distract her for the few minutes it's in there.

—ALBERT FINCH, M.D.,
CHILDREN'S HOSPITAL, NORFOLK, VIRGINIA

Once you've removed and read the thermometer, clean it carefully with alcohol so that it is ready for the next use.

THE PITS

Once your child has reached about one and a half to two years old, taking a rectal temperature is usually very difficult. Luckily, doctors say that for children over age one, it's okay to use other methods. Since most kids aren't able to sit still with a thermometer in their mouth for three minutes until they are at least four years old, taking an axillary temperature under the arm is a popular method.

> When taking an axillary temperature, make sure the thermometer is deep in the child's armpit, and that the armpit is "sealed" with the arm tight against the body.
>
> —KENNETH KATZ, M.D.,
> COLUMBIA PRESBYTERIAN MEDICAL CENTER

You can use either a rectal or oral mercury or digital thermometer for this. You'll need to shake the thermometer down below 96 degrees Fahrenheit if it is mercury. Then all you have to do is tuck the end of the thermometer under your child's arm and keep her still for about three minutes.

> When taking an axillary temperature, hold and cuddle your child on your lap to keep him still.
>
> —RUBY ROY, M.D.,
> RONALD MCDONALD CHILDREN'S HOSPITAL
> OF LOYOLA

When reading an axillary temperature, you need to add between one and two degrees to bring it in line with the reading you would get from a rectal temperature. So a reading of 101 degrees Fahrenheit should actually be read as 102 or 103 degrees. Doctors say that this reading, if you consider it along with your child's symptoms, should be accurate enough to help you decide whether to give over-the-counter medication or to call the doctor.

DOWN IN THE MOUTH

When your child is old enough to sit still and hold the thermometer under his tongue without biting down, you can take his temperature orally. This usually happens around age four or five, but "thermometer readiness" varies from child to child.

> Practice with a straw to help your child learn to keep an oral thermometer under his tongue.
> —RUBY ROY, M.D.,
> RONALD MCDONALD CHILDREN'S HOSPITAL
> OF LOYOLA

You'll need a mercury or digital oral thermometer that is clean and ready to go. Shake it down to below 96 degrees Fahrenheit before you start, and then position it way back under your child's tongue.

> Be sure your child hasn't had anything hot or cold to drink for at least fifteen minutes beforehand, as this can change the reading.
> —SUSAN M. MONK, M.D.,
> THE CHILDREN'S MEDICAL CENTER OF DAYTON

Make sure your child is in a comfortable spot, where she can sit still for at least two or three minutes. Provide television, videos, music, or stories as distractions. Any activity that lets your child stay still is fine.

> Use the quickest-reading thermometer you can, have them keep it under their tongue, and let them hold it. Make it a "big boy" or "big girl" thing. Read a story to distract them and keep them still if you need to.
> —MATTHEW O. MCKEEVER, M.D.,
> CHILDREN'S NATIONAL MEDICAL CENTER

Make sure your child doesn't speak or open her mouth while the thermometer is in place. And, of course, make sure she knows not to bite down.

WHEN TO CALL THE DOCTOR

If your child has a fever higher than 104 degrees Fahrenheit, or has a fever you can't bring down with medication, you should contact the doctor, who will probably want to examine her for signs of serious illness. (See "Fever")

You should also seek medical attention or call your nearest poison control center if your child bites down on a mercury thermometer and breaks it. Mercury is highly toxic, and your child will need medical treatment if she has swallowed some.

Tonsillitis

Do you still have your tonsils? There was a time when most people over the age of ten or twelve would say no and recount stories of going to the hospital and coming home to all the ice cream they could eat. But while tonsillectomies are not as common as they once were, tonsillitis is still certainly a problem for many children.

Doctors believe that the tonsils and adenoids are part of the body's immune system. Both of these masses of tissue— the tonsils at the back of the throat and the adenoids high in the throat behind the nose and roof of the mouth—are similar to the lymph nodes or glands found in the neck, groin, and armpits. They hang there at the entrance to the breathing passage and collect germs that are trying to enter the body. They are also thought to help the body develop antibodies that fight germs. Their role apparently gets smaller as kids get bigger, and removing a child's tonsils doesn't seem to impair her ability to fight infection or illness.

Unfortunately, the tonsils and adenoids sometimes become infected by the germs they filter out of the breathing passages and cause problems of their own.

FIRST RESPONSE

IS IT TONSILLITIS?

When the tonsils and adenoids become infected, they can cause throat and ear infections or become so enlarged that they interfere with breathing or swallowing. If your child has the following symptoms, you will probably need to make an appointment with your pediatrician so that the infection can be treated.

Symptoms of tonsillitis:
- Redder-than-normal tonsils
- A white or yellow coating on the tonsils
- A slight voice change due to swelling
- Sore throat
- Uncomfortable or painful swallowing
- Swollen lymph nodes in the neck
- Fever
- Bad breath

Symptoms of enlarged adenoids:
- Breathing through the mouth instead of the nose most of the time
- Nose sounds "blocked" when the person speaks
- Noisy breathing during the day
- Recurrent ear infections
- Snoring at night

- Breathing stops for a few seconds at night during snoring or loud breathing (sleep apnea)

COMFORT CARE

If your child has symptoms of tonsillitis or enlarged adenoids, you can treat any fever, sore throat, or earache he or she might have (see "Earache," "Fever," "Sore Throat"), but the problem will not go away without medical attention. Doctors generally begin by prescribing antibiotics to treat the infection, which could have your child feeling better in a few days.

However, if your child has recurrent infections even after antibiotic treatment, or if he is having trouble sleeping properly (see "Sleep Problems") because his breathing is disrupted by swollen tonsils or adenoids, your doctor might recommend surgery to remove the tonsils, adenoids, or both. Some studies have even shown that removing the adenoids can help some children who have chronic middle ear infections.

> Sometimes a tonsillectomy is a quality-of-life issue. If a child is sick all the time, and it is really impacting the quality of life in the family, it's worth considering even if the child doesn't always have strep infections.
>
> —DAVID CHAIT, M.D.,
> BOYS TOWN NATIONAL RESEARCH HOSPITAL

In fact, despite the fact that treatment with antibiotics is now much more common, doctors still do a fair amount of tonsil removal. These are more often because of upper airway obstruction and sleep apnea than infection, but about 40 percent are still due to sore throats in his practice, says David Chait, M.D., of Boys Town National Research Hospital. Many families, in fact, find tremendous benefit from the surgery.

Occasionally, a particular pediatrician will be categorically opposed to a given procedure, such as tonsillectomy. If your child's pediatrician tells you he's opposed to all tonsillectomies, it might be worth seeking a second opinion. Sometimes if a kid is sick all the time, that in itself is tough on the kid and on the parents. That's another reason to consider tonsillectomy.

Before the surgery, talk with your child's doctor and help explain the procedure to your child. Let your child ask any questions she likes, and try to visit the hospital for a preoperative orientation. (See "Preparing for a Hospital Visit.") Reassure your child that she will not be losing any important parts of her body and that she will not look any different after the operation.

WHEN TO CALL THE DOCTOR

After surgery, a minor amount of sore throat and difficulty swallowing is normal. However, if your child is in a great deal of pain and has such difficulty swallowing that he cannot eat or drink, call your doctor. You should also call the doctor if your child experiences vomiting, fever, or ear pain. If your child experiences bleeding from the nose or throat, his surgeon should be notified immediately.

Tooth Trouble

Even before we can see them, teeth can be a source of pain for our kids. As those first teeth push their way through the gums, they cause more than a little discomfort. If they aren't taken care of properly, your child can end up with painful cavities. An accident that causes a broken or knocked-out tooth can also be a trying experience.

FIRST RESPONSE

TOOTHACHE

A toothache is usually caused by a piece of food (often sweet) that is stuck in a cavity. If you can see a hole in the tooth, and it has food in it, use a toothbrush and warm tap water to try to dislodge the food. This should stop the ache because it will stop the acid production. If food is lodged between the teeth, remove it with dental floss. Don't use a toothpick in either case, say dentists, as this can actually do further damage.

Switch your child to a soft diet of foods that are not sweet, cold, or acidic (which cause further irritation) until you can get him to the dentist for treatment.

TOOTH TRAUMA

If your child injures her gums or teeth, she should be evaluated by a dentist. If the tooth is just loose or slightly displaced, it's okay to wait a day or two if you have no choice. Meanwhile, give your child a soft diet of fairly bland foods. Avoid acidic foods that might irritate.

If the injury is severe or your child's tooth is broken or knocked out, he likely needs immediate medical attention. Collect the tooth—or pieces of the tooth—and see your dentist right away. If it's a permanent tooth, make sure you store it carefully, since it can probably be replaced, as described on page 386.

Teething

There's no set time for teething to begin. Babies are born with sucking and mouthing reflexes and seem to gnaw on things almost from birth. Actual teething can begin at any age from three to fourteen months. However, around four months of age is the most common time for the first tooth to emerge.

You can often tell when children are teething because they aren't sleeping as well, and they drool a lot or are more fussy than normal. This is probably because the chewing causes extra saliva to be swallowed and thus puts extra digestive acid into the stomach.

Kids catch lots of bugs while they're teething because they put everything in their mouths, according to Jill S. Reel, M.D., of Boys Town National Research Hospital. That's why there seems to be increased numbers of colds and ear infections among teething kids; they aren't due to teething itself.

You might be able to make your baby feel a little better by massaging her gums, but this won't provide lasting relief. You can also provide things for your baby to chew on, which will work for a bit longer. Chew toys for pets and teething rings are good for your child to chew on, says Dr. Reel, as is any toy appropriate for your child's age. Just make sure that you wash them frequently. It's better not to use teething biscuits, because there is a slim chance that your child will break off a piece small enough to cause choking.

> Rubber dog bones seems to work better than most teething rings. Just boil them first to make sure they're good and clean, then put them in the refrigerator to make them cold. They have a nice long handle, and a big knob on the end that kids like to get their mouths around. They are also thicker than standard teething toys.
>
> —DONALD F. DUPFRON, D.D.S.,
> MATTEL CHILDREN'S HOSPITAL AT UCLA

Don't use ice or put teething rings in the freezer. Remember that the ice or ring doesn't just touch the gums; it touches the tongue, lips, cheek, and fingers. This can cause frostbite. Instead of ice, try a washcloth soaked in cool water.

Don't use alcohol on your child's gums, either (it's an old folk remedy, but your baby could end up swallowing too much), or topical pain relievers. Babies just tend to suck topical pain relievers right off, so they don't provide lasting help. Tylenol or Motrin (for babies over six months of age) are better.

For skin rash caused by teething and drooling, use a warm washcloth to wipe the skin clean, air-dry, and apply a barrier

(continued)

cream of either Vaseline or A and D ointment, especially at nap time. You can use a bib to protect the neck and chest.

Call your doctor if your child isn't eating or sleeping well, has anything more than a mild fever, or has coughing or diarrhea, which would indicate an illness that goes beyond teething.

COMFORT CARE

If your child has a toothache or a broken or knocked-out tooth, she will need to see the dentist fairly soon. While you're taking the necessary steps to get your child into the dentist's chair, try to provide a little comfort.

CAVITY COMFORT

If your child has a toothache, try to distinguish the type of pain. If it is provoked by heat, cold, or sweets, it could be a large cavity. Have your child avoid the offending stimulus and give an over-the-counter analgesic until you can get him to the dentist.

Preventing Decay

Toothache is the terminal stage of a disease process that's been going on for at least a year and a half. During the first year or so, that process is completely reversible, so prevention is key. Keep your child away from sugary fluids as much as possible.

Remember, transitioning your child to a spouted cup is no better than leaving him on the bottle if the cup is filled with sweetened liquid. It has basically the same effect. Breast-feeding presents the same dangers to the teeth as the bottle. Breast milk has even more sugar than cow's milk and can cause decay if parents aren't careful.

—THOMAS H. LARSON, D.D.S., M.S.,
VALLEY CHILDREN'S HOSPITAL,
MADERA, CALIFORNIA

To prevent early decay, gently clean your baby's gums with a gauze pad after each feeding, and begin brushing with a soft brush and plain water as soon as the first tooth erupts. Never allow your child to go to bed with a bottle containing breast milk, formula, or any sweetened liquid. The American Dental Association recommends that your child visit the dentist for the first time before his first birthday.

To brush a young child's teeth, have her sit on one parent's lap with her head tilted back against that parent. The first parent brushes the teeth, while the other parent sits in front, knee to knee with the first, and holds the child's hands.

—MAN WAI NG, D.D.S., M.P.H.,
CHILDREN'S NATIONAL MEDICAL CENTER,
WASHINGTON, D.C.

Brush your child's teeth with plain water at least twice a day until age two. After that, you can begin to use a fluoride toothpaste and teach your child to brush her own teeth. You'll still need to supervise your child's brushing—making sure that he cleans all teeth properly and doesn't swallow the toothpaste—until about age six or seven. Your child should have regular dental checkups twice a year.

While fluoride helps protect your child's teeth against decay, too much of this good thing can actually spoil her smile. The American Academy of Pediatric Dentistry warns that too much fluoride during childhood can cause enamel fluorosis, which can leave white specks or streaks—or even brown markings—on the teeth. This usually happens when

(continued)

the child is using a fluoride supplement and drinking fluoridated water, or swallows fluoridated toothpaste rather than spitting it out.

Talk to your child's dentist, who can help you find out how much fluoride is in the water your child drinks and determine whether your child needs a supplement. You should also make sure your child never uses more than a pea-sized amount of toothpaste when brushing his teeth, and that he spits it out, rather than swallowing it.

If too much fluoride does discolor your child's teeth, the appearance of the teeth can often be improved with esthetic dental techniques.

To help your child floss food out from between the teeth, have her sit on a low chair with her back to you, and tip her head back against you. This way you can

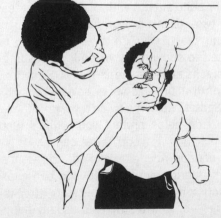

Helping your child floss his teeth.

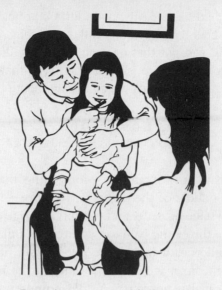

Brushing a young child's teeth.

come from behind and floss as if you were flossing your own teeth.

—MAN WAI NG, D.D.S., M.P.H.,
CHILDREN'S NATIONAL MEDICAL CENTER,
WASHINGTON, D.C.

In a small child, don't use topical anesthetics such as Orajel or oil of clove for toothache, because she could swallow too much of them and get an overdose. Avoid aspirin and Anbesol, too, because they can burn the gums and because aspirin is associated with Reye's syndrome, a potentially fatal complication.

In older children, topical remedies will work only if you have a medium-size cavity and are able to put the drops right on the spot. Avoid icing the area, since cold often makes the pain from a cavity worse.

If your child has a cavity, put a little oil of clove or an over-the-counter preparation with benzocaine on a cotton swab, and put that right on the cavity itself. This will work only if there is actually a cavity that you can see and reach. Oil of clove can irritate mouth tissue, so use it sparingly.

—Donald F. Duperon, D.D.S.,
Mattel Children's Hospital at UCLA

If the pain is spontaneous—something that wakes the child in the middle of the night, for instance—this indicates an advanced stage of decay and possibly damage to the nerve. Sometimes a throbbing pain can come from inflammation of the bone underneath the tooth. You'll often be able to see swelling in the area, which can mean that the root has died and a root canal is necessary. A cold compress or some ice water might soothe the pain; however, if there is a cavity, this will hurt rather than help.

If you see a fiery red area on the gum, about a quarter inch above the tooth, your child likely has a draining abscess. The pain often disappears when the abscess bursts. Your child should see a dentist right away. For either type of toothache you can give Tylenol, but your child should see a dentist as soon as possible for treatment.

MOUTH MISHAPS

Whether you have a teen who plays sports, or a toddler who trips over a toy on the floor, a smack in the mouth often means trauma for the teeth. Because children's bones are soft, baby teeth move more often than breaking in cases of mouth trauma. Permanent teeth are more likely to be chipped.

Prevention of mouth trauma is important. If you have a toddler in the house, do the standard child-safety

things, such as gating off stairways, padding or removing hard edges, and making sure floors are clear and
rugs are secure. If you have a child old enough to play
organized sports, make sure she wears a mouth guard.

—Donald F. Duperon, D.D.S.,
Mattel Children's Hospital at UCLA

Usually, if a toddler has mouth trauma, one of four
things happens:

1. The tooth or teeth are driven back up into the gums.
   In this case, the dentist will wait and evaluate to see
   if the tooth will reerupt; if not it will have to be
   removed.
2. The teeth loosen.
3. The teeth fracture.
4. The teeth are knocked out completely.

In cases of mouth trauma, ice won't help the teeth or
gums. However, it will reduce swelling if the lip is hurt.

These kinds of things almost always involve lip trauma
as well. For any type of mouth trauma, especially in a
toddler, a Popsicle is a great way to keep cold on the
area. The key is to reduce the swelling, which will also
reduce the pain.

—Donald F. Duperon, D.D.S.,
Mattel Children's Hospital at UCLA

After any type of head injury, look for signs of possible
concussion or brain injury (see "Bruises and Black Eyes").
Did your child lose consciousness? Is he alert? Does he
remember what happened? Does he know his name, what
day it is, or similar information? Is he vomiting? Can he focus
his eyes? Are the pupils the same size? If your child shows any

signs of brain injury, don't take him to the dentist; first take him to the emergency room to be treated for the head injury.

Chipping In

If your child fractures a tooth and you can see red or pink, the dental pulp has been exposed. Call the dentist immediately, and try to get to her office as soon as possible. Most children's hospitals and many community hospitals have pediatric dentists on call twenty-four hours a day. You might not need to be seen right away, but the dentist can ask the proper questions to help determine whether it is necessary.

If the chip is significant, find and save the fragment if possible: Just rinse it off and drop it in a glass of water or milk. It can often be bonded back into place, which looks better cosmetically than dental composite.

If a tooth is broken or chipped but you don't see red, your child has probably just fractured the enamel. This can usually be repaired with bonding and a dental composite. You may be able to wait until the next day to see the dentist, but you should still call right away for an evaluation.

A Real Knockout

If your child knocks out a tooth, find it and bring it to the dentist if at all possible. If it's a baby tooth, there's no need for any special treatment, since the dentist won't try to reimplant it. However, she still needs to see it so she can tell whether or not the entire tooth has been knocked out. If a piece of the root is missing, it might have to be removed.

If your child knocks out a permanent tooth and you're able to get to a dentist quickly enough, there's a good chance it can be saved, though this does require special handling. The periodontal ligament cells on the outside of the root need to survive. These are even more important than the nerve at the center of the tooth, since that will likely be removed by root canal anyway. To keep the cells alive, avoid touching the root of the tooth, and keep it wet. Handle it only by the top.

> If a tooth is knocked out, if possible, the first thing to do is put it back where it came from. If the tooth is visibly dirty, rinse it off in tap water first. If it isn't, don't rinse it at all. It doesn't have to be sterile. You can pack the tooth into place with gauze and have your child bite down, or just have her hold it in place with her finger.
>
> —Thomas H. Larson, D.D.S., M.D.,
> Valley Children's Hospital,
> Madera, California

If the tooth is knocked onto a clean surface, rinse it gently with saline solution or milk. If the tooth is dirty and the dirt doesn't come off with very gentle rinsing, swab it carefully with a cotton swab, but don't scrub. Again, the best thing to do is put the tooth back in its socket; but if your child isn't calm enough to keep from swallowing it, or you don't feel comfortable "reinstalling" it, put it in ice–cold milk (ideally, pack the container in ice). That should save it reasonably well for about two hours, until you can get to the dentist. If the tooth is broken, place the pieces in ice–cold milk and bring them to the dentist.

> If you don't have milk, you can put the tooth in saline (such as contact-lens solution), saliva (in your own mouth), or water—in that order.
>
> —Man Wai Ng, D.D.S., M.P.H.,
> Children's National Medical Center,
> Washington, D.C.

To reimplant the tooth, the dentist will first clean it, then position it and splint it with a flexible splint. This will stay on for seven days. After the splint comes off, the child will often need a root canal.

If the tooth has been knocked out of the socket, the five-year survival rate is 20 to 50 percent. Replacement is still practical if the child doesn't yet have all his permanent teeth and is too young for other permanent options, such as bridging. The tooth can be saved long enough for the child to grow into these procedures and to preserve the proper spacing between the teeth.

WHEN TO CALL THE DOCTOR

If your child has a toothache along with signs of systemic infection, such as fever, lethargy, or facial swelling, go to the emergency room or call your pediatrician right away. Also seek immediate medical attention if your child has a severe mouth injury.

If your child has had a filling or minor repair and has pain, swelling, fever, or other signs of systemic infection, call your dentist. Call your doctor as well if your child has a mouth injury that isn't healing within five to seven days.

Urinary Tract Infections

Urinary tract infections (UTIs) are one of the most common serious bacterial infections of childhood, found in 4 to 7 percent of children. They are caused by bacteria that enter the bladder by traveling up through the urethra, the passage that carries urine from the bladder out of the body. These bacteria, often E. coli, usually come from fecal matter. When they invade urine that is held in the bladder, the bacteria have a chance to grow and infect the urinary tract.

If the infection remains in the bladder, this is a lower urinary tract infection. If it continues climbing up into the kidney, it creates an upper urinary tract or kidney infection, which is more serious.

In children, there are three main reasons that urine stays in the bladder rather than being emptied out of the body. Some kids hold their urine too long, or they don't empty the

Boys and Girls

In infancy, boys are more likely to get UTIs than girls, especially those who are uncircumcised. Doctors say that this is no reason to encourage circumcision, because the increased risk is small and is confined to infancy.

After infancy, UTIs are more common in girls, who have a shorter urethra. This means that any bacteria present have a shorter distance to travel to reach the bladder and kidneys.

bladder completely when they go to the bathroom. Obstruction of the bladder can also trap urine, and this can be caused by either constipation (see "Constipation") or congenital abnormalities of the urinary tract.

FIRST RESPONSE

INFECTION DETECTION

In infants, the symptoms of bladder infection are many of the same you would expect to see with any illness. They include fussiness, decreased activity, poor feeding, fever, jaundice, vomiting and diarrhea, and possibly smelly or cloudy urine. There are often no other symptoms.

Kidney infections in the youngest patients also have non-specific symptoms and are difficult to detect. The baby might appear sicker and have a higher fever. Doctors usually have to assume the worst-case scenario when treating infants with UTIs, and treat them like kidney infections. However, UTIs in infants are often missed because people don't check for them.

Parents are most likely to notice that their older child is going to the bathroom more frequently, or has daytime or nighttime wetting even though she has been potty-trained. In addition to the fever, vomiting, and diarrhea present in infants, older kids can also complain of lower abdominal pain and a burning sensation during urination.

Kidney infections usually have the same symptoms as bladder infections, though the child often appears much sicker than one with a bladder infection. Children with kidney infections might also voice complaints of back pain.

Because urinary tract infections will not clear up without antibiotics—and will only get worse if left untreated—it's important that you see your pediatrician if your child shows signs of a UTI.

COMFORT CARE

Doctors say that there isn't much you can do to ease the painful urination often present with UTIs. Luckily, antibiotics can relieve the symptoms in as little as two days, and there are a few comfort measures you can take. You can also encourage good toileting habits to prevent future infections.

PAIN GOING POTTY

Urinary tract infections put parents and kids in a catch-22. In order to help flush out the urinary tract, and to keep it clear of future infections, children need to empty the bladder frequently. But because the infection often hurts, children are reluctant to go to the bathroom.

While you're waiting the day or two for antibiotics to clear up your child's symptoms, doctors recommend giving him plenty of fluids, so that his urine is less acidic and less irritating to the skin. To help the bladder muscles relax and let go, try a soak in a warm tub. You can even allow very young children to urinate in the tub if this helps. Just make sure that you explain that this is because they are ill, and that they shouldn't do it all the time.

> Warm compresses to the bladder area once or twice a day, Tylenol, and encouraging fluids to dilute the urine can all help with painful urination. In older kids, there is a prescription medication sold under the brand name Pyridium available, but it isn't often used in younger children.
>
> —MICHAEL LAMACCHIA, M.D.,
> ST. JOSEPH'S CHILDREN'S HOSPITAL, NEW JERSEY

Because antibiotics are often prescribed before the urine culture is ready and before the doctor knows exactly what type of bacteria is involved, the medicine may not be effective. Call your doctor if your child's symptoms aren't improving in a day or two, because she might need a different antibiotic.

ENCOURAGING GOOD HABITS

Don't Be a Camel

Because urine that's held in the bladder gives bacteria a place to grow, doctors recommend that you teach your child to empty the bladder at least every two to three hours. "Going to the bathroom is something that parents perceive as dirty. I've had parents tell me proudly, 'Oh, my daughter is a little camel. She can go all day without going to the bathroom.' That always worries me because that's the child who's going to come in with a urinary tract infection," says Marc Cendron, M.D., F.A.A.P., of Children's Hospital at Dartmouth.

To encourage frequent urination, and to dilute the urine so that there is less bacteria present, make sure your child drinks plenty of fluids.

> To teach your child to empty his or her bladder completely, count to five, ten, fifteen, twenty, and have him "keep the water going" until the highest number he can reach.
>
> —MARC CENDRON, M.D., F.A.A.P.,
> CHILDREN'S HOSPITAL AT DARTMOUTH

Some kids, especially preschoolers, don't want to go to the bathroom or to stay long enough to empty the bladder completely because they are playing, watching TV, or doing something fun on the computer. You can usually tell if they make frequent trips to the bathroom but urinate only a tiny bit. If you see your child run in and back out after only ten seconds, ask her to go back in and try again. Teach your child to take her time and relax so that she empties the bladder completely.

> Have your preschooler urinate into a plastic cup or measuring cup that you don't use for anything else. Mark or note the level of urine, and play a game where your child tries to fill the cup "just a little more" each time he urinates.
>
> —GLENDA KARP, M.D.,
> CHILDREN'S HOSPITAL OF THE KING'S DAUGHTERS,
> NORFOLK, VIRGINIA

Doctors say that you can help teach your child to empty her bladder completely by playing some simple games. One of these is to make a game of having your child stop and start the stream of urine. Sometimes kids get so accustomed to urinating just a tiny bit that they forget they can restart the stream if it stops.

Since constipation can also keep the bladder from emptying properly, make sure your child has regular bowel movements. If your child doesn't want to use the bathrooms at school because they're dirty, or if your child's teacher is reluctant to let her go to the bathroom often enough, you might have to work with your pediatrician and the school nurse and teacher to reach an acceptable alternative, such as allowing the child to use a more private teacher's bathroom.

Front to Back

Some people think that improper wiping can increase your child's risk for urinary tract infections. The idea is that wiping the wrong way may move fecal matter and accompanying bacteria closer to the opening of the urethra, where it can make the climb up to the bladder.

Doctors say there's no good scientific data to prove this, and that your chances of contracting a UTI have more to do with how virulent the present bacteria happens to be and how strong your body's defense system is. However, for hygiene reasons, proper wiping should be encouraged. Teach your kids to wipe front to back, especially after a bowel movement.

Bubble bath has also been considered a culprit in urinary tract infections, but doctors say that this is an old wives' tale. Bubble baths might cause external genital irritation, but not UTIs.

> If your son is uncircumcised, teach him to retract his foreskin and wash his penis. Children can start to learn this at the same age they start to learn to wash their hands and brush their teeth. Because most boys have been circumcised, we've lost track of that little bit of hygiene.
>
> —MARC CENDRON, M.D., F.A.A.P.,
> CHILDREN'S HOSPITAL AT DARTMOUTH

Tough Tests

Urinary reflux is a condition that causes urine to flow backward from the bladder toward the kidney, rather than from the bladder out of the body. With simple UTIs that aren't the result of reflux, the main effects are local, including irritation and possible scarring to the bladder, and are not serious. However, in kids who have reflux, especially at high levels with recurrent urinary tract infections, there is danger of scarring to the kidney and decreased kidney function.

Because 25 to 50 percent of children under age eight with a specimen-documented UTI (which means that a good sample was taken and cultured) have urinary reflux, have your doctor check for this if your child has had a documented urinary tract infection. There are five grades of reflux, from ten to five, depending on how far up the urinary tract the reflux travels. Grades one to three are almost always outgrown. Grades four and five sometimes require surgery.

Five to 10 percent of kids with a UTI have a physical abnormality of the urinary tract that will cause recurrent infections.

Even though these tests are unpleasant, it is very important for your child to undergo them. Treating underlying problems can prevent serious health damage later.

—RANDALL ROCKNEY, M.D.,
HASBRO CHILDREN'S HOSPITAL,
PROVIDENCE, RHODE ISLAND

Recurrent UTIs that involve the kidney can cause high blood pressure and decreased kidney function, so it's important that doctors detect any abnormalities and prevent future infections. Most kids with urinary reflux outgrow it but will need a preventive course of antibiotics in the meantime. If your child is placed on long-term antibiotics because of reflux, be compliant so that recurrent infections are prevented.

(continued)

Physical abnormalities of the urinary tract can be treated surgically.

The first test for abnormalities is called a voiding cystourethrogram (VCUG). The bladder is filled with "contrast" material through a catheter, and a radiologist examines the urinary tract by taking X rays as the bladder fills and empties. If done by an experienced technician, the experience isn't usually very uncomfortable. The test is especially necessary for kids under age five, who tend to be more prone to kidney damage if they get a kidney infection. This means that any abnormalities need to be detected right away so that infections can be prevented.

> A VCUG should be done by a pediatrically trained staff. I've had many parents come in with horror stories about tests done by staff who didn't have experience with children. If a pediatric anesthesiologist is available, she might be able to provide some mild sedation for kids who've had trouble with this test in the past, or who are having a difficult time.
>
> —Marc Cendron, M.D., F.A.A.P.,
> Children's Hospital at Dartmouth

> Prepare your child for a VCUG by explaining honestly what she can expect. Have her count, blow, or use other distraction techniques while the catheter is being inserted.
>
> —Michael Lamacchia, M.D.,
> St. Joseph's Children's Hospital,
> New Jersey

Another test that's generally done to check for urinary tract abnormalities is an ultrasound of the kidneys to show if they're enlarged. This is noninvasive and causes no discomfort at all. There is also a test called an Intravenous Pyelogram (IVP), in which a radioactive marker is injected into the vein to check for scarring of the kidney in kids who have had repeated infections. The main discomfort here is from the injection.

WHEN TO CALL THE DOCTOR

Because urinary tract infections will not generally clear up and are likely to get worse without antibiotic treatment, call your doctor any time you suspect that your child has a UTI.

If your child is taking antibiotics for a urinary tract infection and the symptoms are not improving after two days, call the doctor again. If the antibiotic was prescribed before the urine culture results came back, it might not be effective against the specific type of bacteria present in your child's infection; the doctor will need to prescribe a different antibiotic.

While your child is on antibiotics, be alert for any side effects such as rash or upset stomach, and call your doctor if they occur. Make sure you give the full course of antibiotics as directed, and go back for the follow-up urine culture to make sure the infection is completely gone.

Filling a Cup

In order to diagnose a urinary tract infection, your child's doctor will need to take a urine sample, which might be easier said than done. If your child is too young to urinate voluntarily, there are three ways to collect a urine specimen. The doctor can insert a needle through the skin and into the bladder to draw urine, but this is painful and isn't often done. More often, urine is drawn through a catheter.

Catheterization is difficult, and there isn't much you can do to make it easier. If your child needs to be catheterized, you need to understand that this is a necessary part of the evaluation process and try to keep your anxiety low. Then you can hold, support and comfort your child during the procedure.

—MARC CENDRON, M.D., F.A.A.P.,
CHILDREN'S HOSPITAL AT DARTMOUTH

(continued)

Sometimes doctors apply a bag to the outside of the child's body, around the genital area, and wait for the urine to collect. However, because the urine is easily contaminated with bacteria from outside the body, this method can yield a false positive reading.

Start giving your child clear fluids to drink about thirty minutes before the appointment, so that the bladder is full at the right time.

—MICHAEL LAMACCHIA, M.D.,
ST. JOSEPH'S CHILDREN'S HOSPITAL,
NEW JERSEY

If your child can urinate on cue, the doctor will likely enlist your help in collecting a sample. You'll probably be given a sterile cup and an antiseptic wipe. First, you will need to clean your child's genital area, pulling back the foreskin to clean if you have an uncircumcised boy.

Turn on a nearby faucet, or try that old summer-camp trick of putting your child's hand underwater to help him get the urge to urinate. In some cases, if your child is really having trouble, your doctor might send home a kit with you so that you can collect the sample later.

—RANDALL ROCKNEY, M.D.,
HASBRO CHILDREN'S HOSPITAL,
PROVIDENCE, RHODE ISLAND

Then have your child urinate a bit, and collect the specimen midstream. This helps ensure that any bacteria present in the urethra are washed away by the first jet of urine, so that the sample reflects only what is present in the bladder. If you have a girl, have her sit with her legs spread wide, so that the folds of the vagina are open. Be patient and try not to make the situation stressful for your child.

If your child is having trouble urinating, it might help to take a brief walk outside to calm her nerves.

—GLENDA KARP, M.D.,
CHILDREN'S HOSPITAL OF THE KING'S DAUGHTERS,
NORFOLK, VIRGINIA

Preparing for a Hospital Visit

The idea of going to the hospital is frightening for children, and may be even more so for their parents. The best way to combat this fear is by gathering good information on what to expect and making some careful preparations. Your doctor and the hospital staff should be able to help you in making the experience as easy as possible for everyone involved.

WHEN TO GET READY

The timeline for telling a child about an upcoming hospital visit depends on your child's age, developmental level, and his condition, though doctors and child-life specialists say that one day in advance per year of age is a good guideline.

You know your child best and should be aware of his or her coping state. How anxious does he get about things? How much information does he usually need? How does he react to things like going to spend the night with a friend or family member? How did he cope on a previous hospital or doctor visit?

—NAOMI MARTINEZ, C.C.L.S.,
SHANDS HOSPITAL, UNIVERSITY OF FLORIDA

For toddlers or preschoolers, one or two days in advance is best. Children don't have a good sense of time at this age, and can't imagine things like "next week." They also won't be able to remember the information as long, so it's better to explain things closer to the date. For school-age kids, discuss the visit five days to a week in advance, to give them time to think about it and come up with questions. Then follow up to make sure your child's questions get answered.

Your child should be involved in her own health care as much as possible from the earliest age. Parents often underestimate their child's ability to cope.

—JAMES ATKINSON, M.D.,
MATTEL CHILDREN'S HOSPITAL at UCLA

Adolescents need to know about health concerns and upcoming hospitalizations from the beginning; around age twelve to fourteen, he can start making some decisions about his treatment options and should be consulted.

Consider the following when talking to your child about an upcoming hospital visit:

- Will your child be able to remember the information you're sharing until the procedure takes place?
- How does your child best take in information: Verbally? In writing? Through pictures? Through play?

> You don't need to bring up the subject of pain unless
> your child asks about it. Sometimes it's more of a
> parental concern than a concern for the child.
>
> —CATHY ROBINSON-LEARN, CHILD-LIFE SPECIALIST,
> MATTEL CHILDREN'S HOSPITAL AT UCLA

For elective situations, talking with your child should probably start when you see the surgeon for the first time. Prepare her for that consultation by explaining what the problem is that you're concerned about, and that the doctor is going to examine her. The doctor will explain the procedure to you in detail, and your child can be there and ask questions or not, depending on what she's comfortable with. Then follow up at home to make sure your child understood what went on and that you can answer your child's questions.

> Each child is different, so you ultimately have to do
> what you think will work best for your child. Remember
> that kids often know what's happening whether some-
> one has told them or not.
>
> —LORI SCHWEIGHARDT, C.C.S.,
> PHOENIX CHILDREN'S HOSPITAL

No matter what your child's age is, doctors say that it's important to be honest in an age-appropriate way. Giving accurate information is much better than leaving things up to the child's imagination. "People will have a five-year-old diagnosed with a malignancy, and they don't want to tell the child what's wrong," says James Atkinson, M.D., professor of surgery at UCLA. "But the child is going to go in for surgery, and go through chemotherapy, and his hair is going to fall out. It's not reasonable to expect that this child won't notice what's going on with his body."

Time for the Pain

Sometimes children need painful procedures—vaccination shots, blood draws, IVs, stitches, etc.—to make them better or keep them well. These things can be frightening for both parent and child, and your number one priority, unless your child is in a life-threatening situation, is to remain with your child. There is no reason a parent shouldn't be present for injections, blood tests, or even sutures. Your child will feel much less frightened if you are there to comfort him.

For short procedures, prepare your child by explaining that it's going to be painful, but it's going to be short.

—James S. Reilly, Alfred I.
duPont Hospital for Children,
Wilmington, Delaware

Since parents generally know in advance that this type of pain is coming, doctors suggest preparing your child honestly. Talk to your doctor beforehand to find out exactly what will happen. This way your child will know and expect each step and will probably be less afraid. But don't fill your child in too far in advance: If you tell him about a shot well before his appointment, he might be afraid all the way to the doctor's office.

Talk with your child's doctor about using local anesthetics to lessen the pain of some procedures. EMLA cream, which is widely available, uses lidocaine and prilocaine to numb the skin before blood draws or injections, but isn't always offered to patients. It honestly isn't used as much as it should be.

—Steven J. Weisman, M.D.,
Children's Hospital of Wisconsin

For longer procedures such as stitching up a cut or setting a broken bone, there are sedatives that can help children relax. One, called Fentanyl Oralet, even comes in lollipop

(continued)

form. Your child won't know enough to ask for these things, so that's your job.

> A baby might be distracted and comforted by a paci-
> fier or bottle. Older children can clench a fist or
> squeeze a toy or blow. Tailor your distraction to the
> age of the child.
>
> —REBECCA J. PATCHIN, M.D.,
>   RONALD McDONALD CHILDREN'S HOSPITAL
>   OF LOYOLA

When anesthetics aren't available, parents must rely on the time-honored art of distraction to take kids' minds off whatever is hurting them. The old standards, such as reading a book or singing a song, might work. Your child can also develop coping mechanisms to help when she is scared—for instance, when separated from a parent in order to enter the operating room. Your child can often have a comfort item (such as a stuffed animal or blanket) with her. She can also try deep breathing, imagining pleasant things, or listening to music if it is available. Whatever coping method you have practiced, be sure to share it with the medical staff so they can help your child use it.

> Have your child blow bubbles (pack your soap and
> bubble wand) or toot on a party horn. These things
> help focus and relax your child's breathing while giv-
> ing them a pleasant image to concentrate on.
>
> —STEVEN J. WEISMAN, M.D,
>   CHILDREN'S HOSPITAL OF WISCONSIN

Some children, however, prefer to focus on what's happening to them. In this case, explain or ask the medical staff to explain step by step what is going on.

> If you're going to fall apart and really can't be with
> your child through a difficult procedure, that doesn't
> mean you have to be disconnected from what is
> going on.

- Be there with your child when the procedure is explained, so that you know what will happen.
- Tell the person who will be performing the procedure about your child. Share information about past health-care experiences, or things that made the procedure easier if your child has had it before. Explain how your child routinely behaves in similar situations. Does she scream frantically at first and then calm down? Is the procedure easier if he lies on his side? This type of information can help the technician and your child.

—CATHY ROBINSON-LEARN, CHILD-LIFE SPECIALIST,
MATTEL CHILDREN'S HOSPITAL AT UCLA

WHAT KIDS ARE AFRAID OF

Kids have different fears at different ages, and some of them are not what parents expect. Some kids will express their fears openly, while others will not. A parent can sometimes tell their child is anxious by changes in behavior.

Try asking your younger child to draw a picture about going to the hospital, and you might find out his fears. For older children, you can mention some common concerns and talk about issues that "other kids her age" have when they go to the hospital.

—SANDRA DAIGNEAU, B.S., C.C.L.S.,
HASBRO CHILDREN'S HOSPITAL,
PROVIDENCE, RHODE ISLAND

The most common fear in toddlers and preschoolers is being separated from their parents, so reassure your child that you will be with him and that he will get to come home once the visit is over. Preschoolers are often afraid that the hospital visit is a punishment for something they did wrong, so explain that this is not the case. They are also usually afraid of the big machinery (CAT scans, MRI machines, and even X-ray machines).

> Infants, toddlers, and preschoolers will look to you to know how to respond. You need to stay calm.
>
> —LORI SCHWEIGHARDT, C.C.S.,
> PHOENIX CHILDREN'S HOSPITAL

School-age children are concerned about being separated from their parents as well, but they also worry about needles and pain, and about something bad happening to their bodies. Kids this age tend to have a fear of anything unknown, which is why you need to let them ask questions about what will happen. Validate their concerns, explain that everyone is afraid, and give them information about what will happen. Don't tell them to "be brave."

> Be honest about what's going to happen. If your child is going to have a shot and she's had one before, ask her what it felt like the last time.
>
> —CATHY ROBINSON-LEARN, CHILD-LIFE SPECIALIST,
> MATTEL CHILDREN'S HOSPITAL AT UCLA

Kids are often frightened by new people and strange environments: for example, doctors looking at their bodies—especially if they have been taught about "good" and "bad" touch—foreign equipment, or seeing other children who might be very ill and appear different from them (for example, using wheelchairs or IVs). As kids get older, they also tend to think about death, or they might be concerned about how a procedure could change their appearance.

When talking to your child about what will happen, try to be more specific than "This will hurt." Say that a needle might pinch, a cotton swab might feel cold, or that medication might feel warm as it's going into the vein.

—Tiffany Andiloro, C.L.S.,
St. Joseph's Children's Hospital, New Jersey

More mundane concerns among older children include what their routine will be like while they are in the hospital, where their meals will come from, where they will sleep and bathe, and what they will do before and after the procedure.

Children of all ages are somewhat concerned about pain and pain control, so it's important to explain to them that someone will be able to help them if they're in pain.

—Sandra Daigneau, B.S., C.C.L.S.,
Hasbro Children's Hospital,
Providence, Rhode Island

Adolescent children are most often concerned with loss of control, waking up during surgery, and privacy and nudity: They want to know who will see them while they're undressed. Older kids might also be concerned about "sounding like a baby," which often makes them reluctant to mention their pain or fears.

What to Pack

In general, your child can bring to the hospital whatever comfort or luxury items she likes. Depending on the length of the visit, you might even want to bring things to decorate the walls a bit. Here are some things child-life specialists think most kids will want to pack:

- Pacifiers and nipples for bottles for infants
- Pictures of family, friends, and pets
- Favorite music and radio or portable CD player
- Books, puzzles, games, a laptop computer
- Pajamas or extra clothes, especially if it's a longer stay
- Personal hygiene items, including things like nail polish for girls
- Homework or schoolwork, if applicable
- Posters from their room
- Phone numbers of family and friends
- A favorite cup
- Favorite blankets
- Slippers
- Videotapes of the family

If you'll be rooming in with your child, or spending a great deal of time at the hospital, pack a few things for yourself as well, such as extra clothes, personal hygiene items, or anything else you might like to have on hand.

PREPARING YOURSELF

In order to help your child get ready for an upcoming hospital visit or procedure, you'll need to be prepared yourself. Dealing with any fears, concerns, or misconceptions up front will help you keep from passing them along to your child.

The best place to start gathering information is from your child's doctor. He should be able to give you information about your child's condition, and an idea of what to expect. He can often guide you to other good sources of information as well. Nurse specialists who might be working with your child, and child-life specialists at the hospital, can also be of help.

> Ask your doctor to help you evaluate and interpret any information you collect on the Internet. The parent-support groups found these can sometimes be helpful. However, they sometimes attract a larger proportion of people than normal who have experienced complications or side effects connected with a given condition or procedure, so they could give parents the wrong idea or scare them unnecessarily.
>
> —James Atkinson, M.D.,
> Mattel Children's Hospital at UCLA

For more in-depth study, many hospitals offer family resource centers or libraries of information for patients and their parents; these might be accessible on the Internet as well, so don't forget to ask about them. Your local library might be of help, and agencies or organizations devoted to specific conditions—such as the American Heart Association—can provide a wealth of information. If your child's procedure is quite involved, your doctor's office might be able to arrange for you to meet and talk with another family whose child has had the same procedure.

Doctors say that you should understand your child's problem and the purpose of the surgery, the chances that it will help, and any possible side effects and complications. You'll also want to know the exact details of the whole process and what will happen to your child. Are there shots involved? If so how many and what type (skin shots, muscle shots, etc.)?

How might the health-care staff help your child through the experience?

> Find out what your child will look like after the surgery or procedure. Sometimes there are tubes, drains, swelling, casts, or bandaging that might change your child's appearance. It is important to be prepared for this so that you don't overreact when you see your child for the first time after surgery. It is also a good idea for you to know so that you can explain what's going on to your child.
>
> —LORI SCHWEIGHARDT, C.C.S.,
> PHOENIX CHILDREN'S HOSPITAL

Find out when your child needs to stop eating and drinking prior to the procedure. If he's taking medication, find out if he should continue and whether he should bring it to the hospital.

If there will be an incision, learn where it will be, how big it will be, and how long the recovery time will be. Know what to expect from follow-up visits, the purpose of any tubes or drains that will be in place, and when the child will be able to eat again following surgery. What are the pain-control options? What type of home care will be required after the procedure?

> If you're planning to stay with your child, make sure to ask about parking costs at the hospital. It might be worthwhile to have someone drop you off.
>
> —SANDRA DAIGNEAU, B.S., C.C.L.S.,
> HASBRO CHILDREN'S HOSPITAL,
> PROVIDENCE, RHODE ISLAND

If your child will be staying in the hospital, ask how long the hospital stay will be. Get information about rooming-in (staying in the room with your child), visiting hours and rules, what to bring, what food service is available (for parents and kids), and what parking is available and at what cost. Doctors recommend that you make a list of questions and bring it with you when you visit the hospital or your child's doctor prior to the procedure.

PREPARING YOUR CHILD

Taking a tour of the hospital beforehand is the best way for a child to find out what to expect from the minute she walks in the door to the minute she leaves. Call to see about arranging a tour as soon as you find out that your child will be hospitalized. Plan for the preadmission hospital visit to occur shortly after you tell the child about the procedure, but not more than a week beforehand. Younger kids, especially, will forget everything they learned if you visit too early.

> Find out how your child will be put to sleep for surgery. Kids are really concerned about this. Some are more comfortable with an IV, others with a mask. And if you have your child prepared for one thing and then another happens, it will create a lot of anxiety.
> —TIFFANY ANDILORO, C.L.S.,
> ST. JOSEPH'S CHILDREN'S HOSPITAL, NEW JERSEY

> Stress that when a child gets an IV, the needle doesn't stay inside. The needle goes in to guide a tiny, flexible tube that looks and feels like an animal's whisker, but then the needle is removed and just the tube stays in. Many children with IVs are afraid to move because they think they have a needle in their arm.
> —TIFFANY ANDILORO, C.L.S.,
> ST. JOSEPH'S CHILDREN'S HOSPITAL, NEW JERSEY

If the hospital doesn't offer preoperative teaching tours for kids, it still might offer tours for the general public, which would at least help introduce your child to the setting. Ask who might be able to arrange for your child to visit the hospital prior to the procedure. Someone in the pediatrics or social-work department might be willing to help.

On the tour, your child can see most of the parts of the hospital that he will visit (though some tours do not include the operating room) and perhaps receive some hospital items to take home. Your child can play with these items and try them out on a doll. Preschoolers may get a chance to practice putting on the gown, mask, and surgical booties in a non-threatening way that feels like dress-up.

> If your child is going to practice for the hospital, let him decide which stuffed animal or doll he wants to use. Some children are very protective of their stuffed animals and don't want them threatened. If you need to, buy a new stuffed animal for this purpose.
>
> —Lori Schweighardt, C.C.S.,
> Phoenix Children's Hospital

If your child doesn't want to participate much during the hospital tour, don't push her, or you might make the hospital seem like a frightening place. Just stick with the tour and allow your child to hang back and listen. She will pick up plenty of information even if she doesn't appear to be.

If your hospital doesn't offer anything at all for kids, look for books and videos that might have information. You can sometimes borrow teaching materials from your nearest children's hospital even if your child won't be a patient there. Some of these materials are available on-line as well. If you don't have items from the hospital, you can look for a kit at a toy store so your child can engage in medical play. However, don't force the issue if your child doesn't want to play.

If you are planning to teach your child a particular coping or relaxation technique, role-play it as much as possible before the actual procedure. These techniques can
include imagining a favorite place, blowing bubbles,
blowing a feather on a string, reading, or listening to
music.

—NAOMI MARTINEZ, C.C.L.S.,
SHANDS HOSPITAL, UNIVERSITY OF FLORIDA

During the days before the procedure, encourage your
child to talk and express her feelings. This will allow you to
correct any misconceptions she might have about what's
going to happen. If she doesn't want to talk, try having her
draw a picture. This can be especially helpful for younger children who lack the vocabulary to express themselves. Sometimes you might need to talk about your own feelings to help
your child open up. It's fine to let your child know that you
feel nervous about what's going to happen. Then talk about
what you're going to do to make sure that everything goes
okay. To help your child feel more in control at a time when
he might be feeling helpless, give him as many choices as possible and involve him in getting ready for the procedure. Let
him decide what he wants to pack, what he wants to eat the
night before, etc.

If you'll be wearing a surgical gown, put it on at least
one time at home, so that your child can get used to
seeing you that way. You'll be wearing it before and
after your child is in surgery, and you don't want him to
be frightened. Stress that you look funny in the gown,
and that it's okay for him to laugh at you.

—TIFFANY ANDILORO, C.L.S.,
ST. JOSEPH'S CHILDREN'S HOSPITAL, NEW JERSEY

AT THE HOSPITAL

One of the best things to do if your child is in the hospital, according to doctors and child-life specialists, is to be there as much as possible. Many hospitals even offer rooming-in so that you can stay overnight in your child's room. Of course, depending on the length of your child's visit, and your other responsibilities, you might not be able to be there the entire time. Even if you don't have other matters to tend to, you might find that you need a break or some time to yourself, which is just fine. You won't do your child any good if you're not emotionally as well as physically present so that you can give her the attention she needs. Find someone else to stay with your child for a few hours if you need to, so that you can have some time off.

> If you have a large family or circle of friends who will want to visit your child, establish your own visiting hours and schedule and let people know about it up front. Often, everyone wants to be there the day the child comes out of surgery, but the child is not feeling well enough for all these visitors. And then days later there are no visitors at all. Set your own limits and spread the flow of visitors out to cover the entire hospital stay.
>
> —Sandra Daigneau, B.S., C.C.L.S.,
> Hasbro Children's Hospital,
> Providence, Rhode Island

Ask about staff who can stay with your child; many hospitals have volunteers who come in for that purpose. You might also ask family members or friends to stay with your child when you can't. If you're going to be gone just a short while, your child might watch a video with the promise that you will be back when the video is over. If you have a baby or young toddler in the hospital, leave an audiotape of yourself reading, singing, or talking to your child. The staff can play this by the bedside.

> If you have to leave an infant, leave a piece of clothing or a blanket with your scent on it.
>
> —Naomi Martinez, C.C.L.S.,
> Shands Children's Hospital,
> University of Florida

> If your child cannot eat, don't eat in front of her. Go somewhere else to eat.
>
> —Tiffany Andiloro, C.L.S.,
> St. Joseph's Children's Hospital, New Jersey

If you have to leave, never sneak out. Let your child know you're leaving and when you'll be back, then make sure you're back at that time so you don't damage your child's trust. Give the hospital staff the phone number where you can be reached in case your child wants to call you. If you're gone for a long time, call to let your child know you're thinking of him.

> Make a sign for your child's room that answers the following questions:
>
> - What does your child like to be called?
> - What time does your child generally go to bed and wake up?
> - What foods does your child like and dislike?
> - What are your child's security or transitional objects?
> - What other things should the staff know about your child?
>
> —Sandra Daigneau, B.S., C.C.L.S.,
> Hasbro Children's Hospital,
> Providence, Rhode Island

To make things easier for both your child and the hospital, let the staff know what your child likes—food, toys, videos, etc. Don't feel like you're imposing if you tell them that your child doesn't like spaghetti. It's better for them to know so they can make your child more comfortable. Also explain about your child's normal schedule, including the bedtime routine. Nighttime is one of the scariest times for a child in the hospital, and if you have to be away, it'll help if the staff can make things as normal as possible for your child.

Encourage your child to be compliant with her treatment, even if that treatment is sometimes difficult, such as taking medication that doesn't taste good or doing physical-therapy exercises that are painful.

—Naomi Martinez, C.C.L.S.,
Shands Children's Hospital,
University of Florida

While you're at the hospital, one of your most important jobs is to be an advocate for your child while still helping and working with the hospital staff. Child-life specialists recommend asking questions if you think something is wrong, and letting the hospital staff know right away what your child needs. Let them know if your child is uncomfortable, because you know your child best. Don't assume that the hospital staff knows everything about your child.

Parents' most common mistake when dealing with the health-care system is expecting too much and making a big deal out of every little thing. The way the nurse has tucked in your child's blanket isn't a big deal. Getting your child pain medication when he needs it is. Choose your battles, and keep in mind that things aren't always perfect.

—Cathy Robinson-Learn, child-life specialist,
Mattel Children's Hospital at UCLA

Sometimes you have to sleuth around for people to help you. Maybe you have to seek out someone in the kitchen to make sure your child gets her favorite snack. If you're having a particular problem, you might need to seek out a child–life specialist or a patient advocate to help you. You could also talk to a nursing supervisor. However, don't assume that one staff member is the only one who can solve your problems. Different staff members have different jobs. Get to know everyone who will be caring for your child so that you can get help right away, rather than waiting for one particular person.

> Having a child in the hospital is a difficult experience. Don't let your own anxieties, fears, anger, and other emotions interfere with people doing their jobs and helping your child get well. Remain focused and part of the team. If there is a complication, be prepared to discuss your feelings with the health-care team so that someone can explain things to you.
>
> —JAMES ATKINSON, M.D.,
> MATTEL CHILDREN'S HOSPITAL AT UCLA

Be very careful about having discussions in front of your child, especially if you're expressing frustration with the hospital or health–care providers. This might frighten your child, who is in their care and helpless to change that. Also, don't talk about your other worries in front of your child—for instance, your other children who are left at home, or your time away from work.

Index

Contact dermatitis, 59
Contagious rashes, 298, 305
Cooley's Anemia Foundation, 25
Cool-mist vaporizer, 148, 194, 195, 302, 352
Cornstarch powders, 222–223
Cortisone cream, 60
Cosmetic deformity, 80
Cough, 190–203
  calling the doctor, 202–203
  causes of, 192
  cough drops, 197–198
  fluids and, 195–197
  suppressants, 198, 199
  syrup solutions, 198–201
  vaporizers and, 194–195
Cow's milk, 32, 133, 178, 381
CPR, 192
Croup, 194, 203
Crutches, 87–88
Crying, colic and, 127–128, 130, 132, 134, 141
Cuts and scrapes, 95, 204–215
  bandaging, 210–212
  bleeding and, 205
  calling the doctor, 214–215
  cleaning, 209–210
  medication for, 212–213
  scabs, 213–214
  stitches and, 206–208

Dairy foods, 178
Dander, 18–20, 43–45
Day care, 154
Decongestants, 154, 155, 243, 327–329, 341, 352
Deer ticks, 290
DEET (diethyltoluamide), 295
Dehydration
  chicken pox and, 125, 126
  congestion and stuffy nose and, 147
  cough and, 195, 196
  diarrhea and, 229–232
  exercise and, 312
  fever and, 257–258, 261

mouth pain and, 115
oral rehydration solutions, 230–232, 258
signs of, 21, 232, 318
vomiting and, 320
Dermabond, 206, 208
Dextromethorphan, 199, 200
Diamond Blackfan Registry, 25
Diaper rash, 216–227
  calling the doctor, 227
  diaper cream and, 217, 223–224
  diaper wipes and, 216, 220–221
  powders and, 222–223
  preventive diapering, 218–220
  soothing skin, 217–218
  types of diapers, 218–220
  yeast infections and, 223, 224–226
Diarrhea, 228–238, 257
  antibiotics and, 233
  calling the doctor, 237–238
  causes of, 232–233
  cleaning skin, 236–237
  cramps and, 236
  definition of, 228
  dehydration and, 229–232
  diet and, 234–236, 321
  fluid intake and, 229–232
  iron supplements and, 28–29
Diet and nutrition
  anemia and, 28, 30–36
  canker sores and fever blisters and, 110–111, 113, 114
  colic and, 132–133
  constipation and, 175–179
  dairy foods, 178
  diarrhea and, 234–236
  fiber in, 175–178
  of nursing mother, 132–133
  sore throat and, 353
Digestive problems, cow's milk and, 32
Digital thermometers, 254, 368, 370, 371
Disposable diapers, 219
Dog ticks, 290–291
Dramamine, 316

Premature babies
  anemia and, 22
  supplements and, 37
Preventive diapering, 218–220
Prickly heat, 299–300
Prick puncture (scratch) allergy
        testing, 14, 15
Primary headache disorder, 271–273
Protein, 178
Pseudophedrine, 155
Psoriasis, 59
Pyridium, 392

Rash, itching, 297–306
  calling the doctor, 304–306
  contagious, 298, 305
  dry skin, 299–302
  impetigo, 74, 298, 303
  poison ivy, oak, and sumac,
        297–299, 303
  scabies, 297–299
Rashes, allergies and, 13
RAST test, 15
Rebound effect, 154
Rebound headaches, 268
Rectal thermometers, 253–254,
        367–370
Red blood cells, 22
Reye's syndrome, 77, 123, 124, 243,
        259, 267, 308, 319, 383
Rice cereal, 235
RICE (rest, ice, compression,
        elevation)
  for bruises, 96–99
  for muscle ache, 309–310
  for sprains and broken bones, 80,
        82
Rid, 280
Ringworm, 297
Robitussin Pediatric Cough
        Suppressant, 199
Rocky Mountain spotted fever, 289,
        290
Root canal, 384, 386, 387
Rotavirus, 232–233
Rubbing-alcohol baths, 256

Salicylic acid (see Aspirin)
Saline nose drops, 149–152, 327,
        352
Salmonella, 233
Salt-water gargle, 353
Saltwater rinses, for canker sores and
        fever blisters, 109, 110
Scabies, 297–299
Scabs, 213–214
Scrapes (see Cuts and scrapes)
Second-degree burns, 103
Sedatives, 139
Seizures, 109, 212, 348
Separation anxiety, 342–343, 405
Septal hematoma, 77, 80
Severe allergic reactions, 18, 21, 288,
        295–296, 305
Sickle cell anemia, 22, 24
Sickle Cell Disease Association of
        America, 25
Sickle Cell Information Center, 25
Sinus headache, 265, 325, 329
Sinusitis, 155, 158, 159, 163,
        323–330
  allergies or colds and, 324–325, 330
  calling the doctor, 329–330
  incidence of, 323
  medication and, 325, 327–328
  symptoms of, 325–326, 329–330
Sitz baths, 217, 236
Sleep, 331–349
  amount of, 348–349
  bedtime routine, 338–340
  calling the doctor, 347–348
  common problems, 341–347
  environment, 335–336
  good sleep habits, 332–334
  headache and, 274–275
  nightmares and night terrors, 335,
        344–347
  pacifiers and, 336–337
  thumb sucking and, 336–337
Sleepwalking, 343–344, 345
Smoking, asthma and, 45
Sneakers, 63
Snoring, 340, 347